Digital Twins

This book centres on the topic of digital twins for superior healthcare decision support, as access is enabled to large volumes of multi-dimensional data such as patient's electronic medical records, medical scans, and data. The reader learns about the possibility of a digital representation of analogous clinical cases built from data-driven models to represent and present relevant information and germane knowledge in context.

Together with cutting-edge technologies, the authors share the ability of data-driven models to offer more efficient clinical decision support. The authors take a three-prong approach in the study of digital twins, the positive contributions made in other industries, the different types of applications and the numerous benefits offered. Artificial intelligence (AI) techniques, such as machine learning (ML) and deep learning (DL) algorithms, are discussed in the context of digital twins in healthcare applications. By looking at digital twins it is possible to reduce workflow challenges and provide fast and precise diagnosis. This then demonstrates how digital twins therefore support superior clinical decision-making. Importantly, the authors identify critical success issues, including co-design and research, for the design, development, and deployment of suitable digital twins.

This book is written for the healthcare audience, professionals, physicians, medical administrators, managers, and IT practitioners. It also serves as a useful reference for senior-level undergraduate students and graduate students in health informatics and public health.

Nilmini Wickramasinghe is the Optus Chair and Professor of Digital Health at La Trobe University. She has been actively researching and teaching within the health informatics/digital health domain. In 2020, she was awarded an Alexander von Humboldt award for her outstanding contribution to digital health.

Nalika Ulapane is a researcher contributing to the design, development, and assessment of digital health solutions. He brings mathematical modelling, engineering systems design, and design science research principles to solve problems in complex systems like the healthcare sector.

Amir Andargoli focuses primarily on digitalization and digital transformation within the healthcare sector. He draws upon principles from information systems and management to conduct his research, which has resulted in publications in peer-reviewed journals and international symposiums.

Analytics and AI for Healthcare

Artificial intelligence (AI) and analytics are increasingly being applied to various healthcare settings. AI and analytics are salient to facilitate better understanding and identifying key insights from healthcare data in many areas of practice and enquiry including at the genomic, individual, hospital, community, and/or population levels. The Chapman and Hall/CRC Press Analytics and AI in Healthcare Series aims to help professionals upskill and leverage the techniques, tools, technologies, and tactics of analytics and AI to achieve better healthcare delivery, access, and outcomes. The series covers all areas of analytics and AI as applied to healthcare. It will look at critical areas including prevention, prediction, diagnosis, treatment, monitoring, rehabilitation, and survivorship.

About the Series Editor

Nilmini Wickramasinghe is Professor of Digital Health and the Deputy Director of the Iverson Health Innovation Research Institute at Swinburne University of Technology, Australia, and is inaugural Professor – Director Health Informatics Management at Epworth HealthCare, Victoria, Australia. She also holds honorary research professor positions at the Peter MacCallum Cancer Centre, Murdoch Children's Research Institute and Northern Health. For over 20 years, Professor Wickramasinghe has been researching and teaching within the health informatics/digital health domain. She was awarded the prestigious Alexander von Humboldt award in recognition of her outstanding contribution to digital health.

Translational Application of Artificial Intelligence in Healthcare – A Textbook
Edited by Sandeep Reddy

Dimensions of Intelligent Analytics for Smart Digital Health Solutions
Edited by Nilmini Wickramasinghe, Freimut Bodendorf and Mathias Kraus

Digital Health: A Primer
Nilmini Wickramasinghe

Using Blockchain Technology in Healthcare Settings: Empowering Patients with Trustworthy Data
Edited by Ben Othman Soufiene, Saurav Mallik and Abdulatif Alabdulatif

Modern Technologies in Healthcare: AI, Computer Vision, Robotics
Edited by Temitope Emmanuel Komolafe, Patrice Monkam, Blessing Funmi Komolafe and Nizhuan Wang

Scalable Artificial Intelligence for Healthcare: Advancing AI Solutions for Global Health Challenges
Edited by Houneida Sakly, Ramzi Guetari and Naoufel Kraiem

Digital Twins: For Superior Clinical Decision Making
Nilmini Wickramasinghe, Nalika Ulapane and Amir Andargoli

For more information about this series please visit: https://www.routledge.com/analytics-and-ai-for-healthcare/book-series/Aforhealth

Digital Twins
For Superior Clinical
Decision Making

Nilmini Wickramasinghe, Nalika Ulapane,
and Amir Andargoli

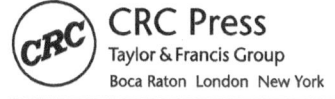

CRC Press
Taylor & Francis Group
Boca Raton London New York

CRC Press is an imprint of the
Taylor & Francis Group, an **informa** business

Designed cover image: Getty Images

First edition published 2026
by CRC Press
2385 NW Executive Center Drive, Suite 320, Boca Raton FL 33431

and by CRC Press
4 Park Square, Milton Park, Abingdon, Oxon, OX14 4RN

CRC Press is an imprint of Taylor & Francis Group, LLC

ISBN: 978-1-032-78035-1 (hbk)
ISBN: 978-1-032-78034-4 (pbk)
ISBN: 978-1-003-48597-1 (ebk)

DOI: 10.1201/9781003485971

Typeset in Palatino
by KnowledgeWorks Global Ltd.

"Innovation distinguishes between

a leader and a follower"

– Steve Jobs

This book is dedicated to our families,

friends, colleagues, and students

and all healthcare stakeholders.

Contents

Part I   The Why of Digital Twins/Why Now

Part II   The What of Digital Twins

Part III   The How of Digital Twins

Foreword

As we enter the second quarter of the 21st century, the promise of the exponentially accelerating power and reach of advanced computing technologies, especially artificial intelligence (AI) which is already yielding unprecedented benefit in almost all aspects of life, is yet to be deployed to achieve the ultimate vision for one of the most important sectors of society – namely, efficient, effective, and optimized healthcare delivery that is tailored to the specific and unique characteristics and health needs of every individual.

However, of all the remarkable advances in AI, the application of digital twins, while yet to be harnessed and applied to their full potential, does offer the most tantalizing and achievable potential to meet that lofty goal.

In this vibrant and highly engaging book, *Digital Twins: For Superior Clinical Decision Making*, by Professor Nilmini Wickramasinghe, Dr Nalika Ulapane, and Dr Amir Andargoli, the authors lay out, in a series of crisply written chapters, the rationale for digital twins in healthcare (the WHY), the characteristics of digital twins best suited to application in healthcare (the WHAT), and exemplar application settings in which digital twins can have the greatest impact (the HOW).

This book not only sets out a strong case and a guide to the evolution, impact, and value of digital twins applied to healthcare, but it also offers signposts to their future evolution, thus providing the reader with literacy regarding both the technology and key emerging use cases for the application of digital twins for the greatest benefit.

This book makes a truly valuable contribution to knowledge. I wholeheartedly recommend it to all healthcare stakeholders.

John Zelcer
La Trobe University

Preface

Today, we are juxtaposed with great technological advances and challenging pressures on healthcare delivery.

On the one hand, technology, especially with respect to computational power, has increased exponentially, but now it is also possible to contain this power in small devices like a wearable device or mobile phone. This, in turn, enables us to make massive strides with analytics, machine learning, and artificial intelligence (AI) most importantly *in situ* in real time. Such capabilities would have made individuals such as Alan Turing, often referred to as the father of AI, tremendously excited in anticipation of what can become possible. In fact, it is only now that ChatGPT is the first form of AI that has passed the Turing test; hence, demonstrated it is not possible to tell definitively if output from ChatGPT is from a human or machine.

On the other hand, we are also experiencing a healthcare delivery crisis at a global level that has never been experienced before. As we have emerged from the 2020 COVID-19 pandemic, we are witnessing tremendous economic pressures, a tired and jaded healthcare workforce, escalating costs to keep everyone stronger for longer, a rapid rise in chronic health conditions such as diabetes and cancer, as well as tremendous increases in various forms of mild to severe mental health issues. Moreover, the existing fatigued healthcare workforce is experiencing high turnover, compressed consulting times and pressure to increase throughput while simultaneously processing ever expanding volumes of multi-spectral data.

Einstein famously noted that to optimally solve problems in a domain it is necessary to look outside the domain. Thus, in this book we proffer the notion of looking outside the healthcare domain, at the opportunities afforded to us by enhanced computational power, advances in analytics, machine learning, and artificial intelligence and looking to digital twins to assist healthcare to cut through the current Gordian Knot and deliver superior care to everyone, everywhere, every time through the use of digital twins, a concept first emerging in the 1960s at NASA.

Our book then, is one of the first to interrogate the case of embracing the construct of digital twins for healthcare contexts. Specifically, it does this by focusing on three key parts: I – The Why of Digital Twins/Why Now, II – The What of Digital Twins, and III – The How of Digital Twins.

Part I: The Why of Digital Twins/Why Now consists of three chapters:

Chapter 1: Decision-Making in Healthcare and the Rise of Technology and the Impact of the Digital Transformation

Chapter 2: Digital Twins in Other Industries

Chapter 3: The Case for Digital Twins for Healthcare

These chapters serve to set the scene and unpack the digital twin construct.

Part II: The What of Digital Twins provides the technical backbone of digital twins and consists of the following four chapters:

Chapter 4: From Algorithms to Outcomes: Leveraging Machine Learning Clustering Techniques for Enhanced Clinical Decision Support

Chapter 5: Clinical Decision Support through Federated Learning and Blockchain

Chapter 6: From Algorithms to Outcomes: Leveraging Machine Learning Classification Techniques for Enhanced Clinical Decision Support

Chapter 7: From Perceptron to Liquid Neural Networks: The Evolution of Neural Networks and Their Role in Black Box Modelling for Digital Twins in Healthcare

Finally, Part III: The How of Digital Twins describes in three key chapters how digital twins can and should be embraced in various healthcare contexts and operations.

Chapter 8: Digital Twins and Clinical Decision-Making

Chapter 9: Application of Digital Twins in Healthcare Processes

Chapter 10: The Impact of Blockchain and Digital Twins in the Pharmaceutical Industry

No one book can ever hope to cover all aspects of any complex construct. But it is our hope that this book will provide awareness of the importance of embracing digital twins for healthcare operations, the imperative to do so and serve as a primer for assisting those who want to design, develop, and deploy digital twins and/or interact with them in clinical contexts. In fact, we contend that AI-empowered digital twins will be as impactful to healthcare delivery as antibiotics were to medicine over 100 years ago. We are confident that as technology continues to advance, digital twins will grow in sophistication and capability, and we encourage all our readers to embrace digital twins for healthcare delivery today to ensure that tomorrow we can deliver world class care every time for everyone everywhere.

Nilmini Wickramasinghe
Nalika Ulapane
Amir Andargoli
Melbourne, January 1, 2025

Part I

The Why of Digital Twins/Why Now

1

Decision-Making in Healthcare and the Rise of Technology and the Impact of the Digital Transformation

Pressures and Challenges in Healthcare Delivery

In order to appreciate the role for digital solutions in healthcare delivery, it is first necessary to understand the unique aspects of the healthcare industry, the key challenges, and the components of the healthcare value proposition (Wickramasinghe & Schaffer, 2010). Unlike most other industries, healthcare has the unique structure that the receiver of the services (i.e. the patient) is often not the predominant payer for those services (i.e. the insurance company) (Wickramasinghe & Schaffer, 2010). Moreover, any healthcare intervention is complex and typically involves directly or indirectly a multiplicity of players including providers, payers, patients, and regulators and what has been noted as the web of players (von Lubitz & Wickramasinghe, 2006) This then leads to many economic dilemmas such as moral hazard, orthogonal considerations pertaining to cost versus quality and information asymmetry which in turn have the potential to create obstacles in an attempt to deliver efficient and effective healthcare (von Lubitz & Wickramasinghe, 2006; Wickramasinghe & Silvers, 2003; Wickramasinghe et al., 2006). In order to ameliorate these problems, relevant data, pertinent information, and germane knowledge play a vital role and can only be obtained via the prudent structure and design of technology (von Lubitz and Wickramaisnghe, 2006; Wickramasinghe & Schaffer, 2010; Wickramasinghe, 2007). Of equal significance are the major challenges facing today's healthcare organizations, i.e., demographic challenges, technology challenges, and finance challenges (Brailer & Terasawa, 2003; Wickramasinghe, 2007).

Demographic challenges are reflected by longer life expectancy and an ageing population; technology challenges include incorporating advances that keep people younger and healthier; and finance challenges are exacerbated by the escalating costs of treating everyone with the latest technologies. Healthcare organizations should respond to these challenges by focusing on three key solution strategies, which taken together form the healthcare value proposition (Wickramasinghe & Schaffer, 2010); namely:

1. access – caring for anyone, anytime, anywhere;
2. quality – offering world class care and establishing integrated information repositories;
3. value – providing effective and efficient healthcare delivery.

These three components are interconnected such that they continually impact on the other and all are necessary to meet the key challenges facing healthcare organizations today. In such a context, it is yet again only through the judicious application of technology solutions that effect superior healthcare delivery (Wickramasinghe & Schaffer, 2010).

Today, the healthcare industry continues to be at the forefront of agendas globally. Between 1970 and 1997 the average percentage of Gross Domestic Product (GDP) on healthcare by members of the Organization for Economic Cooperation and Development (OECD) countries rose from about 5% to roughly 8% (Huber, 1999). Since 2000, total spending on healthcare in these countries has been rising faster than economic growth. Challenges including technological changes, longer life expectancy, and population ageing serve to push health spending up further. Hence, such a growing health spending creates a significant cost pressure for several countries (OECD, 2010a). In 2019, prior to the pandemic, OECD countries spent on average 8.8% of GDP on healthcare, a figure relatively unchanged since 2013 (OECD, 2022). By 2021, this proportion had jumped to 9.7% (OECD, 2022). However, 2022 estimates point to a significant fall to 9.2%, reflecting a reduced need for spending to tackle the pandemic but also the impact of inflation (OECD, 2022).

Reducing these expenditures as well as offering effective and efficient quality healthcare treatment is a priority worldwide. Technology and automation in general have the potential to reduce these costs (Abd Ghani et al., 2010). Moreover, the use of information and communication technologies (ICT) and digital health solutions in particular appears to be the key to respond to these challenges (Wickramasinghe & Schaffer, 2010).

Given that the current situation is no longer feasible, we are witnessing a focus by all OECD countries on developing new healthcare reforms where a key role is played by digital health solutions empowered by artificial intelligence (AI) (Wickramasinghe & Schaffer, 2010).

Clinical Decision-Making

Decision-making in dynamic and complex environments is quintessential to healthcare delivery and the care pathway or treatment trajectory. Today more than ever, voluminous data and information permeate a physician's clinic or a hospital and processing these data manually has and continues to negatively impact healthcare costs as well as make the healthcare system inefficient and ineffective (Wickramasinghe & Schaffer, 2010). Hence digital solutions which coordinate organizational tasks provide information at the point of care, reduce clinical and/or hospital cost, and support quality healthcare delivery are being embraced (Lenz et al., 2012). Such solutions are now playing a critical role in healthcare delivery because they offer several advantages over manual approaches as follows: (1) *Facilitate delivery of care*: digital health solutions can help deliver care to people who are located in remote areas, and who do not have access to hospitals or clinics. For example, doctors may use telemedicine equipment such as Tele-stetascope, Tele-biologic diagnosis equipment, Tele-radiology, and Tele-surgery to diagnose and treat patients because they provide greater accessibility and availability to healthcare solutions (Hojabri et al., 2012). (2) *Improve quality of care*: digital solutions can help to provide easier, safer, and faster access to patient data including laboratory results, therapeutic procedures, medication administration, clinic notes, and billing. This allows the healthcare professionals to access the right data and information at the right time (Austin & Boxerman, 2003). This results in information-based diagnosis, acceleration of communication, and reduction in medical errors (Szynkiewicz, 2012). Further, computerized physician order entry (CPOE) systems, for example, allow bar code reading to match patients to their prescribed medications (Bernstein, 2007) which in turn can serve to reduce medical errors (Bates, 2000; Ball & Lillis, 2000). (3) *Reduce cost and save time*: digital health solutions can help healthcare professionals to access health information in a timely manner. This reduces the issue of staff shortage as well as increases efficiency. Clinical and administrative costs can be reduced by avoiding the duplication of medical examinations and unnecessary visits. For example, by embracing cloud technology, the Swedish Red Cross was able to save 20% on their IT operating costs. This action led to freeing 25% of people's time to focus on more strategic tasks, better supporting the core missions of the organization (Szynkiewicz, 2012). (4) *Support better management and monitoring*: patients learn how to control and manage their disease correctly with the help of online disease management systems. This is particularly important in the context of chronic diseases. Features like "Ask a physician", web-based nurse line, or call centre assist patients to take control of their disease rather than solely rely on a doctor (Ball & Lillis, 2000). (5) *Provide decision support*: web-based clinical decision support systems can give automatic alerts and warnings to physicians. For example, a community hospital in the USA used a computerized alert system to target 37 drug-specific adverse reactions. They detected opportunities to prevent injury at a rate of 64 per 1000 admissions; 44% of the true positive alerts had not been recognized by the physician (Bates, 2000).

It is useful to understand decision-making in healthcare delivery. Specifically, one can think of this in terms of Churchman's (1971) inquiring organizations who defined five inquiring systems: Leibnizian, Lockean, Hegelian, Kantian, and Singerian (Churchman, 1971). Each of these represents a type of inquiring organization from a system view of knowledge creation, examination, and management (Churchman, 1971; Courtney, 2001).

Table 1.1 summarizes these five types.

TABLE 1.1

Five Types of Inquiring Organizations

Type	Description
Leibnizian inquiring system	Use formal logic and analysis to generate fact nets (Churchman, 1971; Courtney et al., 2005; Hall & Croasdell, 2005). Knowledge creation in this system is limited as it focuses on reliability and replication; therefore they deal with problems that are highly structured with few unknown variables (Courtney et al., 2005; Hall & Croasdell, 2005; Mason & Mitroff, 1973; Parrish Jr & Courtney, 2012). Most suitable for digital solution types of expert systems (Hall & Croasdell, 2005; Mason & Mitroff, 1973; Parrish Jr & Courtney, 2012).
Lockean inquiring system	Contain community members sharing a common language and mindset supported by strong relationships and communication (Courtney, 2001; Hall & Croasdell, 2005; Mason & Mitroff, 1973; Parrish Jr & Courtney, 2012). Knowledge is constructed through observation and discussion; it is shared and perpetuated within the organization through attention to symbolic references such as legends and/or well-respected authorities (Hall & Croasdell, 2005; Mason & Mitroff, 1973; Nonaka et al., 1998; Parrish Jr & Courtney, 2012). Examples of IS/IT(information systems/ information technology) utilizing the Lockean inquiring system include data warehouses (storing observations), data mining (analysing the observations), and groupware tools like emails (facilitating the communication and sharing) (Courtney, 2001).
Singerian inquiring system	Generate cycles of processes which resolves problems and disagreements by introducing new variables and laws to provide guidance and overcome inconsistencies at each cycle, until the problem is fully investigated and understood from all sides (Courtney, 2001; Hall & Croasdell, 2005; Mason & Mitroff, 1973; Parrish Jr & Courtney, 2012). Knowledge must be connected to measurable improvements and is judged not only by organizational standards but also by what is good and ethical for all of society. Singerian organizations considering all forms of knowledge include tacit and explicit, deep and shallow, declarative and procedural, exoteric and esoteric (Hall & Croasdell, 2005; Mason & Mitroff, 1973; Nonaka et al., 1998; Parrish Jr & Courtney, 2012). The Singerian approach is best supported by networks based on groupware and web-based to allow virtual information gathering and learning because of its need to include a wide range of individual stakeholders. Repositories and document management systems are supportive tools for information gathering and dissemination process (Hall & Croasdell, 2005; Mason & Mitroff, 1973; Parrish Jr & Courtney, 2012).

(Continued)

TABLE 1.1 *(Continued)*

Five Types of Inquiring Organizations

Type	Description
Hegelian inquiring system	Builds new synthesis by reflecting and resolving diametrically opposed perspectives. Hegelian organizations have little structure or formal mechanism for guidance; however, it is assisted by group support systems that include negotiation and arbitration (Courtney, 2001; Hall & Croasdell, 2005; Mason & Mitroff, 1973; Parrish Jr & Courtney, 2012). Knowledge is managed by analysing the debate of interaction dialogues and the constructed new theory. IS/IT solutions that support Hegelian inquiring systems include groupware that is designed to support and facilitate arguments among stakeholders in order to help them understand the specific elements of each other's proposals; repositories that hold the debate data, document management software, and/or analysis tools for developing points to support either the thesis or the antithesis (Hall & Croasdell, 2005; Mason & Mitroff, 1973; Parrish Jr & Courtney, 2012).
Kantian inquiring system	Incorporate multiple perspectives and facts to determine models and/or system design to discover and distribute information (Churchman, 1971; Courtney et al., 2005; Hall & Croasdell, 2005). The Kantian inquiring system is focused on flexibility, relationships, organizational development through contingency theory and the best-fit between itself and the environment. Hence it can react quickly and effectively to problems and changes (Courtney, 2001; Hall & Croasdell, 2005; Mason & Mitroff, 1973; Parrish Jr & Courtney, 2012). Examples of IS/IT using Kantian systems are the World Wide Web (www), databases, model management systems, decision support systems, and effective information systems (Hall & Croasdell, 2005; Mason & Mitroff, 1973; Parrish Jr & Courtney, 2012)

Source: James F Courtney (2001).

Rise of Technology Advances – IoT, AI, and Analytics, ML AR, VR, MR, Mobile, Sensors, and Wearables

The Internet of Things (IoT) is a system of wireless, interrelated, and connected digital devices that can collect, send, and store data over a network without requiring human-to-human or human-to-computer interaction (Kelly et al., 2020). Such technologies include sensors and wearable solutions. Further, the promise of IoT is in the form of benefits to streamlining and enhancing healthcare delivery to proactively predict health issues and diagnose, treat, and monitor patients both in and out of the hospital (Kelly et al., 2020). Thus, it is now becoming increasingly important to understand how established and emerging IoT technologies can support health systems to deliver safe and effective care. Table 1.2 presents many of these key technological advances in turn.

In addition, other technology developments that have far-reaching benefits to healthcare delivery include augmented reality, virtual reality and mixed reality as well as mobile platforms. However, arguably the most impactful

TABLE 1.2

Key Terms

Technology	Description
AI	AI has developed exponentially especially with the introduction of generative AI such as ChatGPT. There are opportunities for AI to be harnessed to support superior clinical decision-making as will be unpacked in following chapters
Analytics	Analytics or more precisely data analytics involves the systematic computational analysis of data (Agarwal & Dhar, 2014). Data analytics is useful to enable the discovery, interpretation, and communication of meaningful patterns or can entail applying data patterns towards effective decision-making. This is key for healthcare decision-making and specifically the design of digital twins
AR	Augmented reality superimposes digital elements onto the real world to support enhancing perception of the environment) (Interaction design, 2021). This can be helpful for medical education and training
ML	Machine learning is considered a subset of AI that allows machines to learn and improve from experience without being explicitly programmed (interaction design IBM, 2021). This is also important for healthcare as protocols and contexts are dynamic
MR	Mixed reality combines the virtual and physical worlds, allowing both to interact with each other (Interaction design, 2021). This can be helpful for medical decision-making, education, and training
Mobile	Mobile phones and tablets have revolutionized communication (Ling & Donner, 2013). Moreover, they have enabled more personalized and instantaneous support for patients
Sensors	Sensors are devices that detect changes in the source/environment (Javaid et al., 2022) and thus can be very helpful for monitoring patient recovery or change in status
VR	Virtual reality creates a fully immersive digital environment that replaces the real world (Interaction design, 2021). This can be helpful for medical education and training
Wearables	Wearable technologies include all technologies that are designed to work while being worn on the body (Park & Jayaraman, 2021). This makes them very useful for a myriad of healthcare contexts

area today is the rapid advances in analytics, machine learning, and AI. It is predicted that AI in healthcare delivery today will be as significant a game change as antibiotics was to medicine in 1910.

Digital Transformation

Taken together the advances in digital health technologies are enabling the digital transformation of healthcare. This in turn provides the potential for realizing the vision of world class healthcare delivery for everyone, everywhere every time, the realization of a healthcare value proposition of better access, quality, and value for all that is high quality and patient centred. Given the challenges in today's complex and dynamic healthcare environment this digital transformation affords many opportunities to deliver better care for everyone every time.

The Case for Digital Twins

Given the preceding, what is important is to deliver to the healthcare value proposition of better access, quality, and value is personalization and precision and to better track disease progression so that appropriate preventative measures can be put in place ahead of time to avoid catastrophic events that are, potentially life threatening, unpleasant, and expensive to treat. It is the thesis of this book that digital twins afford us this opportunity.

Digital twins, which are essentially virtual replicas of physical entities, have gained prominence across various industries for their potential to enhance understanding, analysis, and decision-making processes (Wickramasinghe & Ulapane, 2024). In the healthcare sector, digital twins have emerged as powerful tools to model and simulate human physiology, enabling personalized and data-driven approaches to healthcare (Wickramasinghe & Ulapane, 2024). The reminder of this book will discuss the critical aspects of digital twins and why they are so beneficial for healthcare delivery and superior decision-making.

References

Abd Ghani, M. K., Bali, R. K., Naguib, R. N., Marshall, I. M., & Wickramasinghe, N. S. (2010). Critical analysis of the usage of patient demographic and clinical records during doctor-patient consultations: A Malaysian perspective. *International Journal of Healthcare Technology and Management, 11*(1–2), 113–130.

Agarwal, R., & Dhar, V. (September 25, 2014). Editorial—Big data, data science, and analytics: The opportunity and challenge for IS research. *Information Systems Research, 25*(3), 443–448. https://doi.org/10.1287/isre.2014.0546

Ball, M. J., & Lillis, J. C. (2000). Health information systems: Challenges for the 21st century. *AACN Advanced Critical Care, 11*(3), 386–395.

Bates, D. W. (2005). Physicians and ambulatory electronic health records. *Health affairs, 24*(5), 1180–1189.

Bernstein, M. L., McCreless, T., & Cote, M. J. (2007). Five constants of information technology adoption in healthcare. *Hospital Topics, 85*(1), 17–25.

Bernstein, S. L., Aronsky, D., Duseja, R., Epstein, S., Handel, D., Hwang, U., ... & Society for Academic Emergency Medicine, Emergency Department Crowding

Task Force. (2009). The effect of emergency department crowding on clinically oriented outcomes. *Academic Emergency Medicine, 16*(1), 1–10.

Brailer, D. J., & Terasawa, A. B. (2003) Use and adoption of computer-based patient records. California HealthCare Foundation, pp. 1–42.

Chan, E., Tan, M., Xin, J., Sudarsanam, S., & Johnson, D. E. (2010). Interactions between traditional Chinese medicines and Western therapeutics. *Current Opinion in Drug Discovery & Development, 13*(1), 50–65.

Chau, C. F., & Wu, S. H. (2006). The development of regulations of Chinese herbal medicines for both medicinal and food uses. *Trends in Food Science & Technology, 17*(6), 313–323.

Churchman, C. W. (1971). *The design of inquiring systems basic concepts of systems.* NY: Basic Books.

Courtney, J. F. (2001). Decision making and knowledge management in inquiring organizations: Toward a new decision-making paradigm for DSS. *Decision Support Systems, 31*(1), 17–38.

Courtney, J. F., Haynes, J. D., & Paradice, D. B. (2005). *Inquiring organizations: Moving from knowledge management to wisdom.* IGI Global.

Flick, U. (2009). *An introduction to qualitative research.* Sage.

Hojabri, R., Borousan, E., & Manafi, M. (2012). Impact of using telemedicine on knowledge management in healthcare organizations: A case study. *African Journal of Business Management, 6*(4), 1604.

Holmes, D. (2011). UK moves to ensure "access to unlicensed herbal medicines." *The Lancet, 377*(9776), 1479–1480.

Interaction design (2021, September 22). What is machine learning? IBM. https://www.ibm.com/think/topics/machine-learning

Javaid, S., Zeadally, S., Fahim, H., & He, B. (2022). Medical sensors and their integration in wireless body area networks for pervasive healthcare delivery: A review. *IEEE Sensors Journal, 22*(5), 3860–3877.

Kelly, J., Campbell, K., Gong, E., & Scuffham, P. (2020) The internet of things: Impact and implications for health care delivery. *Journal of Medical Internet Research, 22*(11), e20135. https://www.jmir.org/2020/11/e20135. https://doi.org/10.2196/20135

Lenz, R., Peleg, M., & Reichert, M. (2012). Healthcare process support: Achievements, challenges, current research. *International Journal of Knowledge-Based Organizations (IJKBO), 2*(4).

Lin, C. H., Pittayachawan, S., Yang, A. W. H., & Wickramasinghe, N. (2014). Using IS/IT to support the delivery of Chinese medicine: A Chinese medicine clinic management system. *International Journal of Biomedical Engineering and Technology, 16*(3), 223–243.

Lin, C. H., Wei, A., Yang, H., Pittayachawan, S., Vogel, D., & Wickramasinghe, N. (2015). *Inquiring knowledge management systems – A Chinese medicine perspective.* Paper presented at the System Sciences (HICSS), 2015 48th Hawaii International Conference on System Science.

Ling, R., & Donner, J. (2013). *Mobile communication.* John Wiley & Sons.

Mason, R. O., & Mitroff, I. I. (1973). A program for research on management information systems. *Management Science, 19*(5), 475–487.

Nonaka, I., Reinmoeller, P., & Senoo, D. (1998). The 'ART' of knowledge: Systems to capitalize on market knowledge. *European Management Journal, 16*(6), 673–684.

OECD (2022) Report available at https://www.oecd.org/en/topics/policy-issues/health-spending-and-financial-sustainability.html

Park, S., & Jayaraman, S. (2021). Wearables: Fundamentals, advancements, and a roadmap for the future. In *Wearable sensors* (pp. 3–27). Academic Press.

Parrish, J. L. Jr, & Courtney, J. F. (2012). Inquiring systems: Theoretical foundations for current and future information systems. In Y. Dwivedi, M. Wade, & S. Schneberger (Eds.), *Information systems theory* (pp. 387–396). Springer.

Qiao, X., Hou, T., Zhang, W., Guo, S., & Xu, X. (2002). A 3D structure database of components from Chinese traditional medicinal herbs. *Journal of Chemical Information and Computer Sciences, 42*(3), 481–489.

Szynkiewicz, P., Iltchev, P., Piechota, A., Sierocka, A., & Marczak, M. (2014). Diagnosis-related groups (DRG) and hospital business performance management. *Studies in Logic, Grammar and Rhetoric, 39*(52).

TCM-ID. (2015). Traditional Chinese medicine information database. http://tcm.cz3.nus.edu.sg/group/tcm-id/tcmid_ns.asp. Traditional Chinese medicine information database. Retrieved 23 December 2015 from Department of Computational Science, National University of Singapore. http://tcm.cz3.nus.edu.sg/group/tcm-id/tcmid_ns.asp

von Lubitz, D., & Wickramasinghe, N. (2006). "Healthcare and technology: The doctrine of networkcentric healthcare" with D von Lubitz Intl. *Journal of Electronic Healthcare (IJEH), 4*, 322–344.

WHO. (2013). *WHO traditional medicine strategy: 2014–2023*. World Health Organization.

Wickramasinghe, N. (2007). Fostering knowledge assets in healthcare with the KMI model. *International Journal of Management and Enterprise Development (IJMED), 4*(1), 52–65.

Wickramasinghe, N., & Schaffer, J. (2010). *Realizing value driven patient centric healthcare through technology*. IBM Center for The Business of Government.

Wickramasinghe, N., & Silvers, J. B. 2003 IS/IT The Prescription to enable medical group practices to manage managed care. *Health Care Management Science, 6*(2), 75–86.

Wickramasinghe, N., Ulapane, N. et al. (2024). Omics-based digital twins for personalised paediatric healthcare. *Studies in Health Technology and Informatics, 24*(318), 180–181. IOS Press. https://ebooks.iospress.nl/doi/10.3233/SHTI240917

Xue, C. C., & O'Brien, K. A. (2003). Modalities of Chinese medicine. In *A comprehensive guide to Chinese medicine*. World Scientific Publishing Co.

Xue, Y., Liang, H., Boulton, W. R., & Snyder, C. A. (2005). ERP implementation failures in China: Case studies with implications for ERP vendors. *International Journal of Production Economics, 97*(3), 279–295.

Yang, A. W., Allan, G., Li, C. G., & Xue, C. C. (2009). Effective application of knowledge management in evidence-based Chinese medicine: A case study. *Evidence Based Complementary and Alternative Medicine, 6*(3), 393–398. https://doi.org/10.1093/ecam/nem124

Zhao, Y., Tsutsui, T., Endo, A., Minato, K., & Takahashi, T. (1994). Design and development of an expert system to assist diagnosis and treatment of chronic hepatitis using traditional Chinese medicine. *Informatics for Health and Social Care, 19*(1), 37–45.

2

Digital Twins in Other Industries

Introduction

Digital twin (DT) technology has evolved from a theoretical framework into a transformative tool with widespread applications across diverse industries. Initially pioneered by NASA during the Apollo missions for troubleshooting spacecraft, the concept gained prominence in the manufacturing and aerospace sectors, where it provided virtual replicas of physical systems for real-time monitoring, simulation, and optimization. Over time, advancements in technologies such as the Internet of Things (IoT), artificial intelligence (AI), and data analytics have enabled DTs to become integral to various other industries, including construction, energy, retail, and urban planning.

Today, DTs are not merely confined to their early use cases but are revolutionizing multiple sectors by enabling organizations to enhance efficiency, innovate processes, and improve decision-making. These virtual models, which mirror the behaviour and conditions of physical assets, allow industries to address complex challenges such as real-time monitoring, system optimization, and predictive maintenance. By integrating real-world data, DTs facilitate more dynamic, data-driven approaches to solving industry-specific problems.

This chapter explores the application of DTs in industries outside healthcare, such as manufacturing, energy, construction, and retail. It highlights how this technology is reshaping these sectors, improving operational efficiency, fostering innovation, and creating new business opportunities. Each industry faces unique challenges, and DT technology offers tailored solutions that push the boundaries of what is achievable in the digital age.

Background and Origin of Digital Twins

The idea of creating a twin system for monitoring and troubleshooting physical assets originated during NASA's Apollo programme in the 1960s, when physical replicas of spacecraft were kept on Earth to simulate and manage issues experienced in space (Van der Valk et al., 2020). These physical replicas laid the groundwork for the modern DT concept, which formalized in 2003 by Michael Grieves during a lecture on product life cycle management (PLM) at the University of Michigan (Grieves, 2014). Grieves (2014) proposed

---

                                                              DOI: 10.1201/9781003485971-3

that a DT consists of three main components: the physical entity, the virtual entity, and the data connection between them. This conceptual framework allowed for real-time data exchange between the physical and digital entities, enabling continuous monitoring and analysis.

NASA's interest in the DT concept intensified as they realized its potential for mission-critical systems, particularly in aerospace applications where simulation and predictive capabilities could reduce risks and improve mission success (Shafto et al., 2010). The transition from physical replicas to digital counterparts was fuelled by advancements in sensor technology, the IoT, and machine learning, all of which allowed for the seamless integration of real-world data into digital models. The realization of DT systems has been significantly enhanced by key technologies such as data-driven modelling, smart sensing, machine vision, extended reality, database techniques, data mining, and scalable cloud and edge computing, all of which enable real-time decision-making, efficient data management, and immersive human-machine interactions (Friederich et al., 2022; Jiang et al., 2021; Knebel et al., 2023; Rasor et al., 2021; Shao et al., 2023).

Definitions of Digital Twins

Although the definition of a DT has evolved over time, there is still no single universally accepted standard (Sharma et al., 2022), with many definitions being presented depending on the context of their application (Schleich et al., 2017). One widely referenced definition comes from Glaessgen and Stargel (2012, p. 7), who described the DT in the context of Aeronautics and space as "an integrated multiphysics, multiscale, probabilistic simulation of an as-built vehicle or system that uses the best available physical models, sensor updates, fleet history, etc., to mirror the life of its corresponding flying twin". This definition emphasizes the role of DTs in mirroring the behaviour of complex systems by integrating data from multiple sources and scales. Similarly, Grieves and Vickers (2017, p. 94) defined a DT as "a set of virtual information constructs that fully describes a potential or actual physical manufactured product from the micro atomic level to the macro geometrical level". The idea revolves around creating a digital informational construct that mirrors the physical system, with a constant flow of data between the two throughout the entire life cycle (Grieves & Vickers, 2017).

Digital Twins in Manufacturing

Manufacturing faces many issues, such as frequently changing demands, the need for real-time monitoring, increasing system complexity, and pressure to improve cost-effectiveness; DTs help address these challenges by enabling continuous assessment, control, and optimization of production processes (Friederich et al., 2022). A DT in manufacturing, as defined by ISO 23247, is a " is a fit for purpose digital representation of an observable manufacturing element with synchronization between the element and its digital representation" (ISO/DIS 23247-1, 2020, p. 3). DTs are one of the main concepts in Industry 4.0 (Masood & Sonntag, 2020). DTs in manufacturing provide a comprehensive, data-driven simulation model of products, processes, or systems. By integrating real-time data from various sources, including sensors and IoT devices, manufacturers efficiently model and control various aspects of manufacturing (Friederich et al., 2022). The real-time nature of DTs allows for continuous monitoring and simulation of the factory's performance, contributing to energy savings and cost reduction (Friederich et al., 2022).

In addition to these operational benefits, DTs offer broader business advantages such as improved product quality, shorter design periods, and the potential for new revenue streams (Stavropoulos & Mourtzis, 2022). They help reduce warranty costs through better monitoring and forecasting of defects, enhancing customer service. Furthermore, DTs support cost-effective production by enabling better design modification, reducing engineering faults, and shortening product lead times (Stavropoulos & Mourtzis, 2022). For manufacturers facing high competition and demand variability, DTs are key to maintaining efficiency and adaptability. DTs also enhance employee safety and operational autonomy by automating dangerous tasks, allowing human workers to focus on innovation (Stavropoulos & Mourtzis, 2022).

Despite these benefits, the absence of a standardized definition, established protocols, and a consistent implementation framework has hindered the widespread adoption of DT technology (Shao et al., 2023).

Digital Twins in the Energy Sector

DTs are transforming the energy sector by offering advanced capabilities to manage, monitor, and optimize energy consumption in real time (Yu et al., 2022). As energy systems become more complex with the integration of renewable resources like wind farms and solar plants, DTs play a critical role in providing virtual replicas of physical assets that allow for predictive maintenance, risk assessment, and operational efficiency. Through the continuous synchronization of real-time data from IoT devices, DTs enable energy companies to predict equipment failures, reduce downtime, and enhance system reliability, ultimately contributing to more sustainable energy production (Lamagna et al., 2021).

In renewable energy, one of the most prominent uses of DTs is in managing wind turbines and solar farms. DTs provide virtual models that are developed to improve turbine safety, reliability, and performance through proactive monitoring and maintenance (Solman et al., 2022). DTs are also increasingly used to optimize offshore wind farm operations, allowing for enhanced monitoring, failure prediction, and efficient maintenance scheduling, reducing both operational costs and downtime (Xia & Zou, 2023). Furthermore, DTs are also instrumental in optimizing energy distribution through smart grids. By simulating energy flow and analysing various scenarios, DTs help utilities balance supply and demand, ensure energy security, predict loads, integrate renewable energy sources efficiently, and prevent outages (Cioara et al., 2022; Onile et al., 2021; Saad et al., 2020). For instance, in smart grid applications, DTs offer real-time insights that help operators adjust energy distribution based on fluctuating demand or potential disruptions (Cioara et al., 2022). Beyond operational benefits, DTs present opportunities for innovation and the development of new business models in the energy sector. For example, they enable the creation of innovative energy services and promote decentralized models, where citizens and energy resources actively participate as prosumers, contributing to grid sustainability (Cioara et al., 2022).

Digital Twins in Construction and Urban Planning

DTs are transforming both the construction and urban planning sectors by enhancing efficiency, safety, and sustainability across various stages of asset development and management. In construction, DTs create real-time digital replicas of physical structures, allowing for continuous monitoring, simulation, and optimization of building processes and operations (Zhang et al., 2022). By integrating technologies like Building Information Modelling (BIM), IoT sensors, and AI-based analytics, DTs provide a dynamic, data-driven approach to managing construction projects, from design through to operation and maintenance (Zhang et al., 2022). This has resulted in improved decision-making, reduced costs, and enhanced collaboration between stakeholders, leading to better project outcomes.

In urban planning, DTs have emerged as a critical tool for city management, offering a virtual representation of entire cities, neighbourhoods, or infrastructure systems that assist in creation of secure and sustainable cities (Ferré-Bigorra et al., 2022). These urban DTs allow planners to simulate various development scenarios, optimize energy and resource usage, and improve public services such as transportation and utilities (Alva et al., 2022; Boccardo et al., 2024). By enabling real-time data exchange between the physical and digital environments, DTs facilitate better-informed decisions, which are essential for managing complex urban ecosystems (Piras et al., 2024). DTs also support participatory planning processes, enabling citizens to engage with city planning efforts and contribute to decision-making through digital platforms (White et al., 2021). One of the key applications of DTs in urban environments is the simulation of infrastructure systems, including transportation networks, telecommunications, water management, and energy distribution (Callcut et al., 2021). This helps cities enhance sustainability and resilience, while reducing costs and inefficiencies (Hämäläinen, 2021). By enabling simulations of urban environments, DTs assist cities in optimizing urban metabolism and identifying sustainable solutions for addressing climate change and environmental challenges (Hämäläinen, 2021). However, while the benefits of DTs in urban and construction contexts are substantial, challenges remain. DTs offer significant potential in urban and construction contexts, but face several challenges. Data integration and interoperability issues are prominent, with disparate semantic standards hindering seamless collaboration (Lei et al., 2023; Omrany et al., 2023). The lack of standardized protocols and a unified framework for DT implementation is also a major obstacle (Nour El-Din et al., 2022). Cybersecurity concerns, particularly regarding data privacy and protection, are critical challenges that need addressing (Omrany et al., 2023; Zheng et al., 2024). Other significant issues include data accuracy and completeness, scalability and complexity, and the absence of widely accepted standards and governance frameworks (Omrany et al., 2023). The slow pace of digitization in the architecture, engineering, and construction industry further hampers widespread DT adoption (Nour El-Din et al., 2022). Addressing these challenges requires prioritizing standardized data formats, exploring semantic data modelling, implementing robust data governance, and developing comprehensive data protection measures (Omrany et al., 2023). Overcoming these barriers is essential for the broader adoption of DTs across the construction and urban planning industries, where they are poised to become integral components of future smart cities and sustainable development initiatives.

Digital Twins in Retail Industry

DTs are revolutionizing retail by creating virtual representations of stores, products, and customer behaviour. These models enable retailers to optimize operations and enhance customer experiences. In apparel retail, fitting rooms are a critical touchpoint where customer decisions are made. However, underutilized or inefficient fitting rooms can result in missed sales opportunities. DTs can monitor fitting room usage, tracking items brought in and whether those items are purchased. This allows retailers to optimize fitting room availability and improve customer service by notifying staff when customers need assistance (Maizi & Bendavid, 2021; Maizi et al., 2019). Further, virtual fitting rooms (VFRs) powered by DTs allow customers to try on clothes virtually, influencing purchase intentions through psychological factors like rehearsability, sense of ownership control, and self-efficacy (Chung & Tan, 2025). With the rapid growth of online shopping, VFRs represent a key strategy for bridging the gap between online and in-store experiences, helping retailers to reduce return rates and increase customer satisfaction. In addition to VFRs, semantic DTs (semDTs) have proven instrumental in optimizing in-store logistics and improving customer support. By integrating diverse data sources, including real-time sensor data and historical sales information, semDTs provide an enhanced view of product replenishment processes and customer preferences (Kümpel et al., 2021). Retailers use semDTs to visualize store layouts and monitor stock levels, ensuring that shelves are always adequately stocked with popular items. For example, in fast-moving retail environments like grocery stores or fashion outlets, semDTs can predict when products need to be replenished based on past sales trends and current customer activity. A particularly innovative use case is the deployment of semDTs with robotic shopping assistants. These robots use semDTs to provide personalized recommendations, dynamically generating queries that take into account customer preferences and store conditions (Kümpel et al., 2023). For instance, a robot might help a customer find toothpaste from a specific brand that includes natural ingredients, based on real-time inventory data. These robotic assistants can also navigate crowded or changing store environments, making shopping more convenient and efficient for customers (Kümpel et al., 2023). Further, AI and IoT Integration in DTs is playing a transformative role in both customer-facing and back-end operations (Shekhawat, 2023). For instance, cashierless checkouts, computer-vision shelf scanning, and dynamic inventory tracking are helping retailers reduce overhead costs and streamline customer service (Shekhawat, 2023). These systems rely on the convergence of AI and IoT technologies (AIoT), which enable real-time data analysis and machine learning models to predict customer behaviour and optimize store layouts. DTs enable retailers to test various store layouts and product placement strategies. For example, a DT can simulate different store configurations to determine which layout leads to the highest customer engagement and sales (Maizi & Bendavid, 2021; Maizi et al., 2019). Retailers like Walmart have been pioneering the use of AIoT through their DT systems, which help design, test, and deploy innovative customer experiences while increasing store efficiency (Shekhawat, 2023). Also, retailers can also use DTs to analyse customer behaviour, both online and in-store. DTs can dynamically track customer behaviour using real-time data from various sources, enabling more effective product recommendations (Vijayakumar, 2020). This technology also allows businesses to monitor social media engagement, personalize customer experiences, and optimize marketing strategies (Das, 2023). In loyalty schemes, DTs can simulate purchasing scenarios and explore "what-if" situations to improve commercial performance, customer well-being, and sustainability (Battye et al., 2023). While DTs show promise in revolutionizing retail strategies, challenges remain in data accuracy and privacy protection (Das, 2023). As the technology evolves, it is expected to offer greater opportunities for optimization and innovation in retail operations and customer engagement.

Conclusion

DT technology has emerged as a transformative force across various industries, revolutionizing the way businesses manage, monitor, and optimize operations. From its origins in aerospace and manufacturing, DTs have expanded their reach into sectors such as energy, construction, and retail, offering innovative solutions to complex challenges. By creating virtual replicas of physical systems, DTs provide real-time insights that drive efficiency, enhance decision-making, and support predictive maintenance.

In industries like energy and construction, DTs are not only improving operational performance but also facilitating the development of sustainable, data-driven strategies. They enable organizations to simulate different scenarios, optimize resources, and create decentralized, adaptive business models. In retail, DTs are transforming customer experiences and operational logistics by offering real-time insights into store layouts, customer behaviour, and inventory management.

However, challenges such as the lack of standardized frameworks and data integration hurdles remain. Overcoming these obstacles will be crucial for the broader adoption and scalability of DTs. As industries continue to invest in digital transformation, the potential for DTs to enhance operational excellence, foster innovation, and enable sustainable development will only grow. With the continuous evolution of IoT, AI, and data analytics, DTs are poised to play an increasingly central role in shaping the future of multiple industries.

References

Alva, P., Biljecki, F., & Stouffs, R. (2022). Use cases for district-scale urban digital twins. *The International Archives of the Photogrammetry, Remote Sensing and Spatial Information Sciences, 48*, 5–12.

Battye, J., Baudains, P., & Ward, J. A. (2023). *Case Study: Developing a digital twin of a retail loyalty scheme.* Consumer Data Research Centre. Retrieved 25 September 2024 from https://www.cdrc.ac.uk/case-study-developing-a-digital-twin-of-a-retail-loyalty-scheme/

Boccardo, P., La Riccia, L., & Yadav, Y. (2024). Urban echoes: Exploring the dynamic realities of cities through digital twins. *Land, 13*(5), 635.

Callcut, M., Cerceau Agliozzo, J.-P., Varga, L., & McMillan, L. (2021). Digital twins in civil infrastructure systems. *Sustainability, 13*(20), 11549.

Chung, K. C., & Tan, P. J. B. (2025). Artificial intelligence and internet of things to improve smart hospitality services. *Internet of Things, 31*, 101544. https://doi. org/10.1016/j.iot.2025.101544

Cioara, T., Anghel, I., Antal, M., Salomie, I., Antal, C., & Gabriel Ioan, A. (2021). An overview of Digital Twins application domains in smart energy grid. https:// doi.org/10.48550/arXiv.2104.07904.

Das, S. (2023, April 23). Digital twins: the key to unlocking industry 4.0 and beyond. https://doi.org/10.2139/ssrn.4426592

Ferré-Bigorra, J., Casals, M., & Gangolells, M. (2022). The adoption of urban digital twins. *Cities, 131*, 103905.

Friederich, J., Francis, D. P., Lazarova-Molnar, S., & Mohamed, N. (2022). A framework for data-driven digital twins of smart manufacturing systems. *Computers in Industry, 136*, 103586.

Glaessgen, E., & Stargel, D. (2012). The digital twin paradigm for future NASA and US Air Force vehicles. 53rd AIAA/ASME/ASCE/AHS/ASC structures, structural dynamics and materials conference. 20th AIAA/ASME/AHS adaptive structures conference 14th AIAA. https://arc.aiaa.org/doi/10.2514/6.2012-1818

Grieves, M. (2014). Digital twin: Manufacturing excellence through virtual factory replication. *White Paper, 1*(2014), 1–7.

Grieves, M., & Vickers, J. (2017). Digital twin: Mitigating unpredictable, undesirable emergent behavior in complex systems. In *Transdisciplinary perspectives on complex systems* (pp. 85–113). Springer.

Hämäläinen, M. (2021). Urban development with dynamic digital twins in Helsinki city. *IET Smart Cities, 3*(4), 201–210.

ISO/DIS 23247-1. (2020). *Automation systems and integration—Digital twin framework for manufacturing—Part 1: Overview and general principles.* International Organization for Standardization.

Jiang, Y., Yin, S., Li, K., Luo, H., & Kaynak, O. (2021). Industrial applications of digital twins. *Philosophical Transactions of the Royal Society A, 379*(2207), 20200360.

Knebel, F. P., Trevisan, R., do Nascimento, G. S., Abel, M., & Wickboldt, J. A. (2023). A study on cloud and edge computing for the implementation of digital twins in the Oil & Gas industries. *Computers & Industrial Engineering, 182*, 109363.

Kümpel, M., Dech, J., Hawkin, A., & Beetz, M. (2023). Robotic shopping assistance for everyone: Dynamic query generation on a semantic digital twin as a basis for autonomous shopping assistance. Proceedings of the 2023 International Conference on Autonomous Agents and Multiagent Systems.

Kümpel, M., Mueller, C. A., & Beetz, M. (2021). Semantic digital twins for retail logistics. In *Dynamics in logistics: Twenty-five years of interdisciplinary logistics research in Bremen, Germany* (pp. 129–153). Springer International Publishing Cham.

Lamagna, M., Groppi, D., Nezhad, M. M., & Piras, G. (2021). A comprehensive review on digital twins for smart energy management system. *International Journal of Energy Production and Management, 6*(4), 323–334.

Lei, B., Janssen, P., Stoter, J., & Biljecki, F. (2023). Challenges of urban digital twins: A systematic review and a Delphi expert survey. *Automation in Construction, 147*, 104716.

Maizi, Y., & Bendavid, Y. (2021). Building a digital twin for IoT smart stores: A case in retail and apparel industry. *International Journal of Simulation and Process Modelling, 16*(2), 147–160.

Maizi, Y., Bendavid, Y., & Ortmann, J. (2019). Leveraging on the digital twin for improving retail store daily operations management. Proceedings of the 18th International Conference on Modelling and Applied Simulation (MAS).

Masood, T., & Sonntag, P. (2020). Industry 4.0: Adoption challenges and benefits for SMEs. *Computers in Industry, 121*, 103261. https://doi.org/10.1016/j.compind.2020.103261

Nour El-Din, M., Pereira, P. F., Poças Martins, J., & Ramos, N. M. (2022). Digital twins for construction assets using BIM standard specifications. *Buildings, 12*(12), 2155.

Omrany, H., Al-Obaidi, K. M., Husain, A., & Ghaffarianhoseini, A. (2023). Digital twins in the construction industry: A comprehensive review of current implementations, enabling technologies, and future directions. *Sustainability, 15*(14), 10908.

Onile, A. E., Machlev, R., Petlenkov, E., Levron, Y., & Belikov, J. (2021). Uses of the digital twins concept for energy services, intelligent recommendation systems, and demand side management: A review. *Energy Reports, 7*, 997–1015.

Piras, G., Agostinelli, S., & Muzi, F. (2024). Digital twin framework for built environment: A review of key enablers. *Energies, 17*(2), 436.

Rasor, R., Göllner, D., Bernijazov, R., Kaiser, L., & Dumitrescu, R. (2021). Towards collaborative life cycle specification of digital twins in manufacturing value chains. *Procedia CIRP, 98*, 229–234.

Saad, A., Faddel, S., Youssef, T., & Mohammed, O. A. (2020). On the implementation of IoT-based digital twin for networked microgrids resiliency against cyber attacks. *IEEE Transactions on Smart Grid, 11*(6), 5138–5150.

Schleich, B., Anwer, N., Mathieu, L., & Wartzack, S. (2017). Shaping the digital twin for design and production engineering. *CIRP Annals, 66*(1), 141–144.

Shafto, M., Conroy, M., Doyle, R., Glaessgen, E., Kemp, C., LeMoigne, J., & Wang, L. (2010). Draft modeling, simulation, information technology & processing roadmap. *Technology Area, 11*, 1–32.

Shao, G., Hightower, J., & Schindel, W. (2023). Credibility consideration for digital twins in manufacturing. *Manufacturing Letters, 35*, 24–28.

Sharma, A., Kosasih, E., Zhang, J., Brintrup, A., & Calinescu, A. (2022). Digital twins: State of the art theory and practice, challenges, and open research questions. *Journal of Industrial Information Integration, 30*, 100383. https://doi.org/10.1016/j.jii.2022.100383

Shekhawat, S. (2023). Making retail smarter with digital twins. *ITNOW, 65*(2), 56–57.

Solman, H., Kirkegaard, J. K., Smits, M., Van Vliet, B., & Bush, S. (2022). Digital twinning as an act of governance in the wind energy sector. *Environmental Science & Policy, 127*, 272–279.

Stavropoulos, P., & Mourtzis, D. (2022). Digital twins in industry 4.0. In D. Mourtzis (Ed.), *Design and operation of production networks for mass personalization in the era of cloud technology* (pp. 277–316). Elsevier. https://doi.org/10.1016/B978-0-12-823657-4.00010-5

Van der Valk, H., Haße, H., Möller, F., Arbter, M., Henning, J.-L., & Otto, B. (2020). A Taxonomy of Digital Twins. 26th Americas Conference on Information Systems.

Vijayakumar, D. S. (2020). Chapter eleven - digital twin in consumer choice modeling. In P. Raj & P. Evangeline (Eds.), *Advances in computers* (Vol. 117, pp. 265–284). Elsevier. https://doi.org/10.1016/bs.adcom.2019.09.010

White, G., Zink, A., Codecá, L., & Clarke, S. (2021). A digital twin smart city for citizen feedback. *Cities, 110*, 103064. https://doi.org/10.1016/j.cities.2020.103064

Xia, J., & Zou, G. (2023). Operation and maintenance optimization of offshore wind farms based on digital twin: A review. *Ocean Engineering, 268*, 113322. https://doi.org/10.1016/j.oceaneng.2022.113322

Yu, W., Patros, P., Young, B., Klinac, E., & Walmsley, T. G. (2022). Energy digital twin technology for industrial energy management: Classification, challenges and future. *Renewable and Sustainable Energy Reviews, 161*, 112407.

Zhang, J., Cheng, J. C., Chen, W., & Chen, K. (2022). Digital twins for construction sites: Concepts, LoD definition, and applications. *Journal of Management in Engineering, 38*(2), 04021094.

Zheng, Y., Li, T., Ma, W., Zheng, J., Li, Z., & Wang, L. (2024). 5-2: Unveiling Privacy Challenges: Big Data-Driven Digital Twins in Smart City Applications. SID Symposium Digest of Technical Papers. 49–52. https://doi.org/10.1002/sdtp.16992

3

The Case for Digital Twins for Healthcare

Introduction

Simply stated a digital twin is a virtual (or digital) copy of a real-world living or non living entity that is as precise as possible [1]. Such digital twins have been revolutionizing all industries in which they have been embraced from manufacturing to space [1]. To date, digital twins have been enthusiastically embraced in some industries such as manufacturing, however, in others namely the service sector, and especially healthcare there is a noted reticence to adopt this technology advancement to enable superior decision-making [1]. Technology advances especially in analytics and artificial intelligence as well as computational power increases have led to more precision in healthcare decision-making [2, 3] and consequently significant benefits to clinical care. Yet, to date, to realize the benefits of such advances and applications to provide overall superior, personalized, individualized focus around care delivery for most patients is still a distant hope. Especially, in the context of chronic conditions; such as, cancer and diabetes (where multiple factors need continuous monitoring and management and where one's genomic profile plays a key and often subtle role) precision and personalization of care pathways is paramount to ultimate clinical outcome success. Moreover, such patients differ in terms of their personal preferences regarding quality versus quantity of life and thus how best their ensuing treatment should be mapped out needs to be planned and structured. To address this key and arguably growing void and troubling patient concern, we contend that incorporating aspects of digital twins holds the key in providing superior, precise, and personalized chronic condition care. Thus, in this chapter, we explore the application of the digital twin concept in the context of patients with chronic conditions such as diabetes, cancer, or dementia and thereby present the case for digital twins in healthcare to support decision-making as well as shed light on the research question:

> How can we apply the concept of digital twins to assist in the provision of personalised and simultaneously precise care for patients with chronic conditions?

In examining how we might leverage digital twins to assist with personalized and precise care, we proceed as follows: first, we review the medical literature and summarize key aspects of how digital twins are being used

DOI: 10.1201/9781003485971-4

currently in the healthcare space. Drawing from lessons in this extant litera-ture, we classify the concept of digital twins into Grey Box, surrogate and Black Box and present an overview of how they are derived and used to support critical aspects around personalized cancer care. We conclude by discussing potential risk factors, challenges, barriers and facilitators that require attention to progress this approach to ensure the best possible qual-ity of personalized cancer care delivery and clinical practice.

Synopsis on the Use of the Term Digital Twin

Arguably, the genesis for digital twins can be traced to the 1970s when NASA was creating mirrored systems, or simulated environments, to monitor unreachable physical spaces (e.g., spacecraft in mission) [1]. These models can be considered preliminary versions of digital twins [1]. Since then, numeri-cal models and computer simulations of varying complexity have gradually been introduced into numerous fields such as engineering, technology, and manufacturing [1].

It was not until 2000 that the digital twin as a formal concept appeared [1, 4]. Since then, the concept has been interpreted and used in various ways [4]. While there are numerous definitions of the concept [1], it is generally agreed that a digital twin must have three major components [4]:

1. a component from the physical world (e.g., an object, a process, a per-son or a phenomenon);

2. a virtual, or a digital representation of the physical component, and

3. a data stream (sometimes referred to as a Digital Thread [1]) connect-ing the physical and virtual components.

From this, over the next decades, digital twins have become well estab-lished and are being used to great benefit in manufacturing for product design and service management, product life prediction, and real-time mon-itoring of equipment [4]. In healthcare, investment, research, development, and adoption of digital twins was later starting in about 2015 [1]. Moreover, unlike the manufacturing sector, the use of digital twins in the healthcare space is still relatively nascent.

Digital Twins in Healthcare

Quintessential to healthcare delivery is the healthcare decision-making pro-cess. This process has two key parts: clinical diagnosis followed by treat-ment. Clinical diagnosis and treatment involve multi-stage steps composed of several elements and also limitations, especially in regard to chronic condition care. Addressing some of those limitations and improving treatment planning is where the introduction of digital twins to support decision-making has the potential to play a valuable role by providing personalized yet simultaneously precise decision support options [3]. To understand how best digital twins can embraced, we first conducted a systematic review of the medical literature. Specifically, this review serves to assist in understanding how the concept of digital twins has been used in the healthcare space to date. Further, this review assists to understand how digital twins might further benefit healthcare delivery in general and specifically with respect to decision support in the context of chronic care conditions. PubMed – a key database source for medical literature – was used for the search. The search was carried out from September 9, 2020 to October 1, 2020.

Among the healthcare-related items listed from this search, there were items relating to medicine and treatment, as well as pharmaceuticals, biotechnology, prosthetics, and computational biology. All items were alluding to, or making use of, the concept of digital twins in some way. However, as the authors' intentions were to focus explicitly on scenarios of treating human patients, the items were narrowed down by specifying "Species: Humans" – a special filter available in the database. Narrowing in this manner resulted in the following eight papers: [2, 3, 5–9, 10].

The abstracts of the listed papers were analysed to evaluate how well each paper aligned with the objective – studying the use of digital twins in healthcare to treat patients. From the abstracts, it was determined that [2, 3, 5–7] were highly relevant. The papers [8–10] were identified to be not quite relevant as they did not explicitly address "treatment of patients". Reference [8] is related to computational biology, focusing on establishing credibility of computational models in biology. Reference [9] revolved around numerical modelling and computational medicine, focusing on model order reduction to create patient-specific mechanical models of the human liver while reference [10] described prototyping and manufacturing three-dimensional coronary arterial phantoms. As a result, papers [8–10] were excluded without further review.

Next, the abstracts of each paper that were initially listed under the keyword "digital twin", but not listed under the "Species: Humans" narrowing, were processed in order to hand pick any relevant works. From these papers, references [11, 12] were found to be relevant. The work of reference [11] describes a unique scenario of using software agent-based digital twins for overall process management in a healthcare facility. Reference [12] describes the use of an in silico digital twin for epicardial augmentation of the failing heart. Taking into account references [11, 12] as well, a full text review was then conducted of the discovered relevant seven papers: [2, 3, 5–7, 11, 12].

The position paper [2] provides an overview of the current status of cardiovascular modelling, the processes required, and some challenges. Developments in physiological modelling, model personalization, model outcome uncertainty, and the role of models in clinical decision support are addressed and "where-next" steps and challenges are discussed.

According to the review paper [7] digital twins can be used for simulation-based training and knowledge sharing purposes. Especially useful for the field of reproductive endocrinology, infertility, and assisted reproductive technologies, and will facilitate teamwork and enable better transmission of knowledge.

A summary of the findings is presented in Table 3.1. The table contains the remainder of the papers that discuss a specific contribution in the form of a digital twin.

Digital Twins for Healthcare

On reviewing the literature, what becomes apparent when considering the use of digital twins in healthcare is that given the complex nature of healthcare operations, it behoves us to categorize or classify specific types of digital twins. In doing so, we have identified three key types as follows:

1. Grey Box digital twins
2. Surrogate digital twins
3. Black Box digital twins

The terms "Grey Box", "Black Box", and "Surrogate" are adopted from the terminology used in systems and mathematical modelling theory [13, 14]. Their meanings, in the context of digital twins, are intended to broadly reflect their standard meaning given in systems and modelling theory. In other words, this terminology indicates that digital twins can be identified as digitally implemented mathematical models. Specifically, based on the characteristics and attributes of the underlying model, we contend that the digital twins can be either Grey Box, Surrogate, or Black Box models (and of course even other classes of models depending on how a premise is defined). A systems and modelling theory perspective to digital twins enables them to be viewed as a mathematical model, which can be useful in formally defining an intended purpose of a digital twin and determine what could possibly (or not) be done with a digital twin – for example a machine learning model can be a mathematical model underpinning a digital twin. The following subsections provide brief summaries to exemplify the meanings of these classifications from the perspective of digital twins and how the reviewed literature maps onto the proposed classification.

Grey Box Digital Twins

A Grey Box digital twin (analogous to Grey Box models [13]) describing a real-world entity, or a phenomenon, would usually have some underlying theoretical model that is well studied and is usually based on some foundational

TABLE 3.1

Summary of Important Papers Uncovered from the Literature Review

Year of Publication	Reference ID	Digital Twin	Focus	Purpose	Way of Use
2019	[5]	Model for vibration of head according to blood flow	Cardiovascular	Diagnosis: detects severity of carotid stenosis	Used to generate data of the vibration of patient's head depending on different degrees of occlusion; best fitting dataset is matched with video of human face; hence approximate severity of carotid artery stenoses is detected
2019	[6]	Model of two-chambered heart with haemodynamic equations and baroreflex-based pressure control	Cardiovascular	Data generation: synthetic photoplethysmogram (PPG) signals	Used to generate synthetic PPG signals for healthy and atherosclerosis condition; can simulate specific "what if" scenarios; can generate synthetic data with pathophysiological interpretability; beneficial for training machine learning algorithms
2019	[12]	Models of heart, the vascular system, and a novel ventricular assist Device (VAD)	Cardiovascular	Treatment planning; dmensioning of novel VAD technologies and future treatment strategies in heart failure	Model is used to: a. confirm in vivo experimental data; b. predict healthy and pathologic ventricular function; and c. assess the beneficial impact of the novel VAD concept
2020	[3]	High-resolution or high-dimensional models of individual patients.	Precision medicine	Treatment planning; precision medicine in terms of identifying best drug regimens for individual patients	Best matching models (i.e., digital twins) for patients are identified from genomic datasets of previous patients. Various drug treatments are simulated on identified digital twins and most suitable regimens are identified based on data
2020	[11]	Agent-based model of the whole trauma care process mimicking a mirror-world paradigm	Trauma management	Better process management and provision of trauma care	Used to enable a trauma leader to continuously monitor the complete state of a trauma (inclusive of prehospital and operative phases, patient, and care team). Trauma lead can have a comprehensive look on an ongoing trauma scenario to make better decisions

science – Physics, for example [13]. For such a model to be complete and serve an intended purpose, it would have to be calibrated to be reflective of a particular instance of the real-world entity or phenomenon. When applied to healthcare, such scenarios can be viewed through an example as follows: think of having a digitally implementable generic model of the human heart with blood vessels that is well studied and validated (such as in [12] for example) – this is a Grey Box model. But, if that model is to mimic the heart and vessels of a particular human, then such a model would have to be calibrated (or tuned) to match the specific human. This calibration may involve some parameter tuning, some estimation, some measurement taking, some data interfacing, and perhaps some human-computer interfacing. On doing so, if the generic model goes on to mimic the behaviour of the heart and vessels of the particular human, then that model becomes a digital twin of the heart of that human. Now, since constructing this digital twin involved some Grey Box identification, we classify this as a Grey Box digital twin. From the works summarized in Table 3.1, [5, 6, 12] are examples of this. Thus, in a healthcare context a digital twin of an organ such as the heart or lungs would be appropriate as a grey box digital twin. In this context, the clinician compares the ideal functioning of the organ as determined by medical science with that of the presenting patient's heart or lung. Then clear care pathways can be identified and decisions made that serve to try to make the presenting patient's heart or lung function more like the desired state.

Surrogate Digital Twins

Surrogate digital twins (analogous to Surrogate models [14]), in the context of healthcare applications, can be considered to be those that are representative of overall processes, or process flows in healthcare facilities (such as in [11] for example). These models would be defined for very specific requirements – for example, an indicator on a computer screen showing in real time the location of an ambulance and the clinical state of its patient to the receiving trauma care facility [11]. This indicator is a part of a digital twin representative of the trauma management process, helping a trauma centre to coordinate ambulance care and trauma centre care. Such digital twins that may not be based on any theory but are constructed to be representative of process flows are the ones we have classified as Surrogate digital twins. Reference [11] is an example. Thus, in the healthcare context, a surrogate digital twin is typically a digital twin of a process such as the ambulance going to the emergency room (ER) and identifying the best process for the patient on arrival at the ER so that vital seconds are not wasted and the appropriate care can be administered.

Black Box Digital Twins

Black Box digital twins (analogous to Black Box models [14]) are those that are neither reliant on well-studied theoretical models such as in the Grey

Box case, nor are defined for specific representative purposes such as in the Surrogate case. In the healthcare context, such digital twins are discovered from data [4] within a model-free paradigm, or a less model-intensive paradigm (as conceptualized in [3] and examined in [4] for example). Principles of probabilistic and statistical learning could play a key role in the construction of these digital twins. In this context, these twins will rely on rich sets of (electronic) medical records of past patients [3]. In principle, when a new patient is presented, a digital twin that matches best to the patient would be able to be discovered from available datasets of previous patients [3]. This approach to data-driven discovery can be envisioned as a way to create digital twins to enhance personalized treatment relevant to personalized cancer treatment planning. In the event of large datasets such as genomic data [3] having to be incorporated – which may be particularly relevant for tasks like cancer treatment planning – using Black Box methods in partnership with advancements in machine learning may be an appropriate way forward. We proffer that this approach of data-driven discovery of Black Box digital twins is a viable way to introduce digital twins to support personalized chronic care planning.

Incorporating Digital Twins in Personalized Chronic Condition Care

In order to understand why we prefer the use of Black Box digital twins for personalized chronic care treatment planning it is necessary to first understand key issues pertinent to chronic care today.

Current Issues in Chronic Care Management

Chronic conditions represent a significant burden on healthcare systems worldwide, with their management posing ongoing challenges [15]. Traditional approaches to chronic care management often lack a person-centered focus, which fails to adequately address the complex needs of individuals with multiple chronic conditions [16]. Furthermore, conventional diagnosis and treatment methods may have limitations in accurately predicting disease progression and optimizing therapeutic interventions [17, 18]. In light of these challenges, the integration of digital twin technology into personalized chronic condition care presents a promising avenue for enhancing patient outcomes and healthcare delivery. Chronic conditions, such as diabetes, dementia, cardiovascular disease, and respiratory disorders, are characterized by long duration and persistent effects on health. These conditions often require ongoing medical attention and management to prevent complications and optimize quality of life.

However, several issues hinder the effective management of chronic conditions within healthcare systems. One of the primary challenges in managing chronic diseases is the presence of comorbidities [19]. This necessitates patients with chronic conditions to seek care from multiple providers across various settings [20], which often results in fragmented care delivery and inadequate care coordination. This fragmentation can lead to communication gaps, redundant services, inconsistencies in treatment approaches, and, consequently, medical errors [18]. Further, traditional models of chronic care management tend to be reactive, focusing on treating symptoms or exacerbations rather than preventing disease progression or addressing underlying risk factors [21]. This approach may result in suboptimal outcomes and increased healthcare costs. Moreover, conventional approaches to chronic care often rely on standardized treatment guidelines that may not account for individual variations in disease presentation, response to treatment, and lifestyle factors [16, 22]. This is very important as conventional diagnostic tests and treatment protocols are often based on population averages and may not take into account individual variability in disease pathology, genetics, and lifestyle factors [23]. This one-size-fits-all approach may lead to disparities in care and ineffective management of chronic conditions [24]. Hence, there exists a compelling necessity for a paradigm shift from reactive to proactive and predictive care, with the goal of administering the appropriate treatment to the right patient at the right time [25]. Digital twin technology has emerged as a novel approach to personalized chronic condition care by generating virtual replicas of individual patients and their physiological systems to address these challenges.

Conventional diagnosis and treatment planning, especially in relation to cancer care, involves a number of key clinical processes [26]. These clinical processes have slowly evolved over many years to manage and guide the best potential outcomes for cancer care in an increasingly complex and diverse knowledge domain. These processes include the following:

1. Clear delineation of anatomical disease site, histopathological type and extent or stage of the disease, which includes capturing demographic data as well as data on relevant patient frailty and comorbidities

2. The treating clinician being familiar with the latest knowledge directly from the medical and scientific literature

3. The latest versions of clinical practice guidelines published by specialist societies relevant to cancer type (e.g., National Comprehensive Cancer Network – NCCN).

4. Evidence from real-world data, e.g., cancer registries

5. Incorporating clinicians' experience, expertise and specific recall of patients from their past experience that may be similar to the patient under care

6. Input to formulating treatment recommendations from all relevant specialists in the context of a multidisciplinary care planning meeting

7. Obtaining patient informed consent about a treatment option, including eliciting patient preferences with respect to quality versus quantity of life

It is useful to note that these seven steps are limited by current diagnostics and processes. Such limitations include [27]:

1. Relying on gold standard clinical trials. Such trials are becoming increasingly problematic as a source of advice due to rapid growth in understanding of cancer biology and available treatment options and the slow and expensive processes involved in the conduct of appropriately powered clinical trials. Stratification of patients in traditional clinical trials according to subgroups that are either predictive of treatment response or of prognosis relevance is becoming increasingly difficult.

2. Clinicians, like all human decision-makers, are probably limited to evaluate 3–5 factors cognitively in making recommendations about patients. However, more recently, massive amounts of information have become available about cancer in general, about the clinical and pathologic course of disease progression for individual patients, and about the factors contributing to individuals' responses to therapeutic regimens which are beyond the cognitive capacity of a clinician or a patient to process in deciding on a treatment option.

3. Substantial heterogeneity of cancer cells and their tumour microenvironment both within a single patient and across patient groups which are nevertheless typically treated as if they were the same, based on traditional criteria. A more granular approach to classification of cancer within these traditional groups is now required to guide effective treatment.

4. Incorporating novel and more effective treatment options requiring data intensive processes, such as identifying genomic alterations (e.g., neurotrophic tyrosine receptor kinase [NTRK] gene fusions) that exist widely across what were previously thought to be unrelated tumour types based on anatomical site of origin (site agnostic).

5. Current approaches to treatment taking insufficient account of patients' preferences and outcomes orientated to those patient-reported outcome measures (PROMs).

6. It has been understood for many years that the evidence base for treating rare cancers is limited because of their rarity and the lack of adequately powered clinical trials to guide treatment recommendations. With a massive increase in data about all cancer patients they are now all rare or unique and require approaches to the formulation of treatment recommendations that reflect that complexity

These identified limitations serve to highlight that the challenges faced in current practices for cancer treatment are primarily concerned with how best to process large, multi-spectral and often disparate data appropriately for a specific context. Identifying strategies to address this challenge, by incorporating digital health solutions to enable and facilitate superior decision support for clinicians, is a key need and a current void; and one for which we contend that the introduction of Black Box digital twins could have the potential to make a preliminary but direct positive impact on improving and personalizing cancer treatment.

In some respects this represents the resurrection, in a different form, of clinical experience which, in recent evidence hierarchies, has been degraded for the obvious reasons that the experience of an individual clinician is limited compared to all available real-word experience, evidence and data. The digital twin concept in some sense expands and formalizes the concept of clinical experience by more exactly matching the current patient to prior patients, and by vastly expanding the number of patient profiles and treatment regimens that can be used to make inferences about the care of the current patient.

A rubric for developing Black Box digital twins for personalized chronic care planning is depicted in Figures 3.1 and 3.2.

Figure 3.2 provides a generic framework about the concept of DTs in healthcare. It depicts the major components of DT stated earlier, which are physical world, digital world and digital threads, and how DT can be utilized in clinical decision support. Figure 3.2 also indicates the three representative

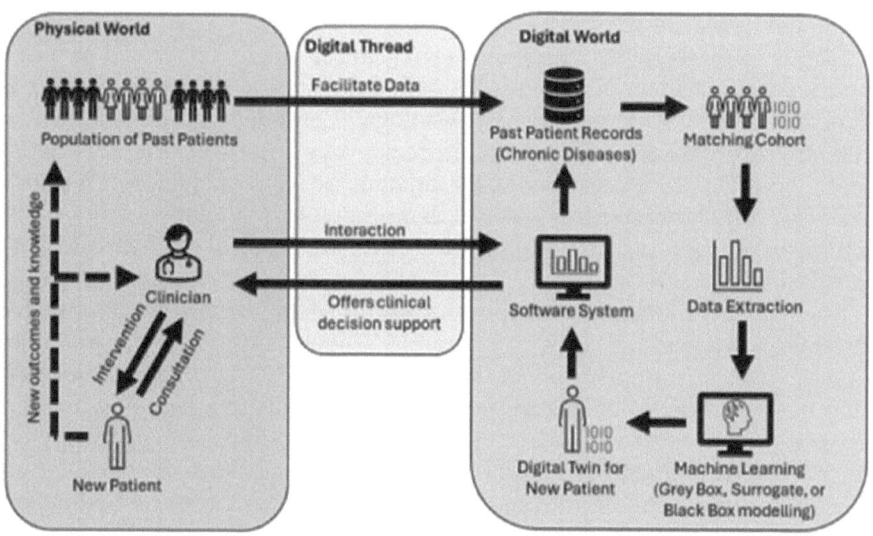

FIGURE 3.1
An overview example for how digital twins operate in healthcare, focused on chronic diseases.

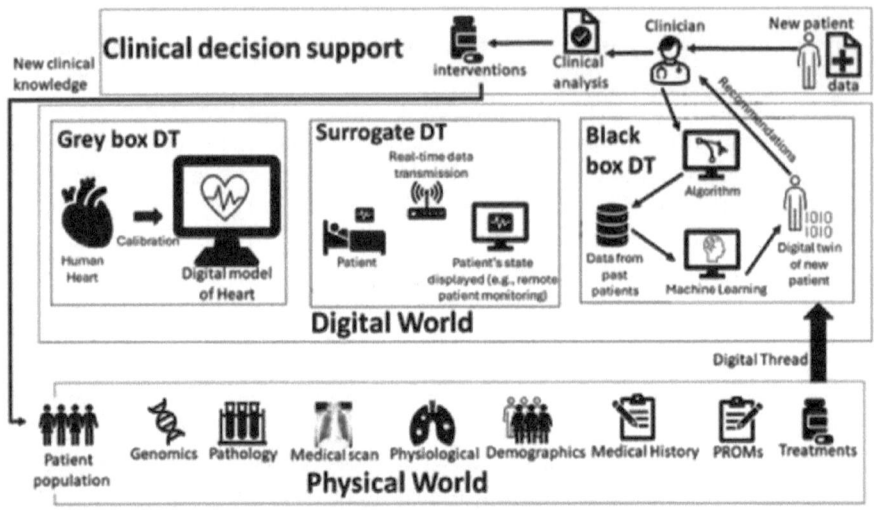

FIGURE 3.2
Types of digital twins and examples for their roles in healthcare.

categories of DT defined in this article, depending on how they are learned at the "Machine Learning" phase. They are components of "Digital Twins World" and are generated from the data stream (i.e. digital thread) from the physical world. The framework is proffered as adoptable for developing digital twins-based solutions to assist personalized cancer care. A more intricated view of how digital twins can be constructed from patients and data is provided in Figure 3.2.

In this framework, uterine endometrial cancer [28] is considered as a case study (as depicted in Black Box DT). There are several influential factors in cancer treatment such as clinical, physiological, and demographic. These factors are captured according to literature surveys and clinicians' knowledge from various data sources (available publicly or from outcomes of randomized controlled trials) such as patient demographics, pathology results, medical history, genomics, physiological information, medical scans, treatments, and PROMs.

The information from these physical world data sources is accumulated to build a database of cases in DT world. They are digital representations of a large patient population in the physical world. The digital representation is also made up of useful prognostic and predictive factors which are ranked and weighted based on evidence such as domain experts' knowledge, clinical reports, and key parameters of AI algorithms for developing the digital twins. AI algorithms are applied to create representative patient populations in the DT repository. Clinicians can use the repository to find the best matched DT model for new data from a real patient and combine clinical experience to identify new interventions. The matched output, the recommended DT, can include information such as matching percentage and treatment suggestions. The identified new clinical knowledge can be further utilized as a new data source in the physical world.

For instance, genomic data is increasingly being widely used for treating endometrial and other cancers [28]. The proffered framework can be used to create digital twins with similarities in genetic and other clinical, histological and chemical pathology data and later can be used to guide treatment of a real patient. When genomic data is used there are enormous variables and interpretations that need to be considered is a mammoth task for clinicians to use to make optimal diagnostic and treatment decisions. By taking advantage of AI algorithms in the proposed framework, clinicians can quickly find the closest similar DT of the patient which will then assist in exploring best potential treatment plans and contribute to optimal decision-making.

Challenges and Risks

As with any technological advancement, the introduction of digital twins to healthcare comes with its own set of issues, risks, and challenges. Critical issues arising when introducing digital solutions to healthcare, such as enterprise-wide Electronic Medical Records, have been noted and documented in the literature. Authors see the same issues becoming relevant for digital twins. The most noticeable issues can be listed as follows: ensuring high standards of performance and fitness of technology for intended purposes [29]; risks of mistakes, and accountability when mistakes happen [30]; Scepticism about Black Box computation, especially among the medical community, and the requirement for explainable artificial intelligence [30]; ethical implications; data security and privacy [30]; legislative challenges and slow adoption of digital solutions in healthcare [30]; and surveillance capitalism [30]. As such, there is opportunity for technologists, clinicians, researchers, ethicists, bureaucrats, legislators, and funders to be aware of the critical issues, and work together to co-design solution and authorizing environments that ensure the best possible quality of healthcare delivery.

Conclusions

The application of digital twins has served to revolutionize key aspects in manufacturing, which in turn has enabled novel and innovative processes to ensue and more personalized and individualized solutions to result. The preceding has served to proffer that similar benefits might ensue in healthcare contexts if the concept of digital twins is embraced, and in some instances expanded or extended, for various healthcare scenarios. We illustrate this vision by discussing the benefits that might be realized to support superior personalized and individualized cancer care planning that would complement advances in precision medicine by augmenting this with findings from psychosocial data, PROMs, as well as cultural and ethnic preferences so that an individual's choice around quantity versus quality of life can also be factored into the clinical decision-making and care planning protocol development. To assist in realizing such a vision for digital twins in healthcare, we identified from our literature review an opportunity to formalize the concept of digital twins in terms of Grey Box, Surrogate and Black Box digital twins for healthcare. Furthermore, we conclude that Black Box digital twin conceptualization is well suited for supporting the delivery of superior personalized and individualized cancer care planning. The opportunity to design and develop digital twins to facilitate clinical decision-making around advanced treatment planning, by coupling with data mining and recent advances in domains such as genome analysis [31], is not only exciting but provides the potential to realize in healthcare, and more specifically cancer care, similar revolutionary advances and benefits as have been enjoyed by manufacturing through its incorporation and application of digital twins.

References

1. Barricelli, B. R., Casiraghi, E., & Fogli, D. (2019). A survey on digital twin: Definitions, characteristics, applications, and design implications. IEEE Access, 7, 167653–167671.
2. Hose, D. R., Lawford, P. V., Huberts, W., Hellevik, L. R., Omholt, S. W., & van de Vosse, F. N. (2019). Cardiovascular models for personalised medicine: Where now and where next? Medical Engineering & Physics, 72, 38–48.
3. Björnsson, B., Borrebaeck, C., Elander, N., Gasslander, T., Gawel, D. R., Gustafsson, M., ... Swedish Digital Twin Consortium (2020). Digital twins to personalize medicine. Genome Medicine, 12, 1–4.
4. Liu, Y., Zhang, L., Yang, Y., Zhou, L., Ren, L., Wang, F., ..., Deen, M. J. (2019). A novel cloud-based framework for the elderly healthcare services using digital twin. IEEE Access, 7, 49088–49101.
5. Chakshu, N. K., Carson, J., Sazonov, I., & Nithiarasu, P. (2019). A semi-active human digital twin model for detecting severity of carotid stenoses from head vibration—A coupled computational mechanics and computer vision method. International Journal for Numerical Methods in Biomedical Engineering, 35(5), e3180.
6. Mazumder, O., Roy, D., Bhattacharya, S., Sinha, A., & Pal, A. (2019, July). Synthetic ppg generation from haemodynamic model with baroreflex autoregulation: a digital twin of cardiovascular system. In 2019 41st Annual International Conference of the IEEE Engineering in Medicine and Biology Society (EMBC) (pp. 5024–5029). IEEE.

7. Ceccaldi, P. F., Pirtea, P., Lemarteleur, V., Poulain, M., Ziegler, D. D., & Ayoubi, J. M. (2019). Simulation and professional development: Added value of 3D modelization in reproductive endocrinology and infertility and assisted reproductive technologies teamwork. Gynecological Endocrinology, 35(7), 559–563.

8. Patterson, E. A., & Whelan, M. P. (2017). A framework to establish credibility of computational models in biology. Progress in Biophysics and Molecular Biology, 129, 13–19.

9. Lauzeral, N., Borzacchiello, D., Kugler, M., George, D., Rémond, Y., Hostettler, A., & Chinesta, F. (2019). A model order reduction approach to create patient-specific mechanical models of human liver in computational medicine applications. Computer Methods and Programs in Biomedicine, 170, 95–106.

10. Renaudin, C. P., Barbier, B., Roriz, R., Revel, D., & Amiel, M. (1994). Coronary arteries: New design for three-dimensional arterial phantoms. Radiology, 190(2), 579–582.

11. Croatti, A., Gabellini, M., Montagna, S., & Ricci, A. (2020). On the integration of agents and digital twins in healthcare. Journal of Medical Systems, 44(9), 161.

12. Hirschvogel, M., Jagschies, L., Maier, A., Wildhirt, S. M., & Gee, M. W. (2019). An in silico twin for epicardial augmentation of the failing heart. International Journal for Numerical Methods in Biomedical Engineering, 35(10), e3233.

13. Tulleken, H. J. (1993). Grey-box modelling and identification using physical knowledge and Bayesian techniques. Automatica, 29(2), 285–308.

14. Müller, J., Shoemaker, C. A., & Piché, R. (2013). SO-MI: A surrogate model algorithm for computationally expensive nonlinear mixed-integer black-box global optimization problems. Computers & Operations Research, 40(5), 1383–1400.

15. Muka, T., Imo, D., Jaspers, L., Colpani, V., Chaker, L., van der Lee, S. J., …, Franco, O. H. (2015). The global impact of non-communicable diseases on healthcare spending and national income: A systematic review. European Journal of Epidemiology, 30, 251–277.

16. Sobolewska, A., Byrne, A. L., Harvey, C. L., Willis, E., Baldwin, A., McLellan, S., & Heard, D. (2020). Person-centred rhetoric in chronic care: A review of health policies. Journal of Health Organization and Management, 34(2), 123–143.

17. Andargoli, A. E., Ulapane, N., Nguyen, T. A., Shuakat, N., Zelcer, J., & Wickramasinghe, N. (2024). Intelligent decision support systems for dementia care: A scoping review. Artificial Intelligence in Medicine, 102815.

18. Brunner-La Rocca, H. P., Fleischhacker, L., Golubnitschaja, O., Heemskerk, F., Helms, T., Hoedemakers, T., …, Zippel-Schultz, B. (2016). Challenges in personalised management of chronic diseases—Heart failure as prominent example to advance the care process. EPMA Journal, 7, 1–9.

19. García-Olmos, L., Salvador, C. H., Alberquilla, A., Lora, D., Carmona, M., Garcia-Sagredo, P., …, García-López, F. (2012). Comorbidity patterns in patients with chronic diseases in general practice. PloS One, 7(2), e32141.

20. Edwards, N. (2012). Improving hospitals and health services delivery: a report on the priorities for strengthening the hospital and health services delivery in the WHO European Region. In Improving hospitals and health services delivery: a report on the priorities for strengthening the hospital and health services delivery in the WHO European Region. https://iris.who.int/bitstream/handle/10665/272465/9789241513906-eng.pdf

21. Glasgow, R. E., Tracy Orleans, C., Wagner, E. H., Curry, S. J., & Solberg, L. I. (2001). Does the chronic care model serve also as a template for improving prevention? The Milbank Quarterly, 79(4), 579–612.

22. Van der Heide, I., Snoeijs, S., Quattrini, S., Struckmann, V., Hujala, A., Schellevis, F., & Rijken, M. (2018). Patient-centeredness of integrated care programs for people with multimorbidity. Results from the European ICARE4EU project. Health Policy, 122(1), 36–43.

23. Horwitz, R. I., Charlson, M. E., & Singer, B. H. (2018). Medicine based evidence and personalized care of patients. European Journal of Clinical Investigation, 48(7), e12945.

24. Barrett, M., Boyne, J., Brandts, J., Brunner-La Rocca, H. P., De Maesschalck, L., De Wit, K., …, Zippel-Schultz, B. (2019). Artificial intelligence supported patient self-care in chronic heart failure: A paradigm shift from reactive to predictive, preventive and personalised care. Epma Journal, 10, 445–464.

25. Bernardini, M. (2021). Machine Learning approaches in Predictive Medicine using Electronic Health Records data (Doctoral dissertation, Università Politecnica delle Marche).

26. Siegel, R., Naishadham, D., Jemal, A. et al. (2013) Global cancer statistics. CA: A Cancer Journal for Clinicians, 63(1), 11–30.

27. Morris, A. M., Rhoads, K. F., Stain, S. C., & Birkmeyer, J. D. (2010). Understanding racial disparities in cancer treatment and outcomes. Journal of the American College of Surgeons, 211(1), 105–113.

28. Dörk, T., Hillemanns, P., Tempfer, C., Breu, J., & Fleisch, M. C. (2020). Genetic susceptibility to endometrial cancer: Risk factors and clinical management. Cancers, 12(9), 2407.

29. Zarinabad, N., Meeus, E. M., Manias, K., Foster, K., & Peet, A. (2018). Automated modular magnetic resonance imaging clinical decision support system (miror): An application in pediatric cancer diagnosis. JMIR Medical Informatics, 6(2), e30.

30. Shaw, J., Rudzicz, F., Jamieson, T., & Goldfarb, A. (2019). Artificial intelligence and the implementation challenge. Journal of Medical Internet Research, 21(7), e3659.

31. Mohanty, R. P., Gamaarachchi, H., Lambert, A., & Parameswaran, S. (2019). Swaram: Portable energy and cost efficient embedded system for genomic processing. ACM Transactions on Embedded Computing Systems (TECS), 18(5s), 1–24.

Part II

The What of Digital Twins

4

From Algorithms to Outcomes: Leveraging Machine Learning Clustering Techniques for Enhanced Clinical Decision Support

Introduction

Clinical decision-making is fundamental for healthcare. It involves healthcare professionals assessing patient data to inform diagnoses and treatment choices. Accuracy in clinical decision-making is crucial for optimal patient outcomes and effective healthcare delivery. However, clinical decision-making encounters several challenges. Cognitive biases, for instance, is one challenge. It can lead to errors in judgements made by clinicians. This becomes so because clinicians may rely on heuristics that do not always align with evidence-based practices. Information overload is another challenge. This challenge arises because of the sheer volume of data that must be analysed by clinicians. Analysing vast amounts of data can overwhelm clinicians. This makes it difficult to discern relevant information quickly. Additionally, variability in clinician expertise can also become a challenge. It results in inconsistent decision-making. That too further complicates patient care and potentially leads to suboptimal outcomes. Issues encountered in clinical decision-making are thus multifaceted (Bijani et al., 2021; Watkins, 2020). These issues highlight the need for enhanced decision support for clinicians. Enhanced clinical decision support can assist clinicians to navigate complex clinical scenarios.

Machine learning (ML) is a subset of artificial intelligence (AI). It has emerged as a promising solution that can address some of the above-mentioned challenges encountered in clinical decision-making. Through ML, algorithms can be used to analyse vast and complex datasets. Through this analysis, complex patterns may be identified. These patterns may not be apparent to human clinicians. But through algorithms, such patterns can be discovered through computation. This capability allows for more informed decision-making. ML techniques can process information at a scale and speed that far exceeds human capacity (Wu et al., 2022).

Clustering techniques play a significant role in ML. Clustering is a way of grouping similar data points without predefined labels (Jain, 2010). In healthcare, hidden patterns and relationships within patient data can be uncovered through this technique. This can enhance our understanding about patient populations. Moreover, this can help the development of informed targeted interventions.

This chapter explores various clustering techniques. These techniques are explored particularly regarding their potential as clinical decision support tools. We look at how these techniques can be leveraged to support healthcare practices. Means such as improving diagnostic accuracy, personalizing treatment plans, and streamlining clinical workflows are particularly focused on. Furthermore, opportunities and barriers associated with the implementation of ML techniques in clinical settings are identified and briefly discussed. Thereby we attempt to highlight the transformative impact ML techniques can have on clinical decision-making by answering the research question: How might clustering techniques enhance clinical decision support?

Clustering: An Overview

Clustering involves grouping a set of objects (or data points). This is done in such a way that objects in the same group (or cluster) are more similar to each other than to those in other groups. The similarity between objects is measured by one or more distance metrics, such as Euclidean Distance (Krislock & Wolkowicz, 2012) or Cosine Similarity (Ye, 2011). In the healthcare context, clustering techniques can help uncover distinct groupings from complex datasets about patients and other healthcare contexts. For instance, when a new patient is presented, clustering can help in identifying a cohort of past patients that best matches the present patient. Identifying cohorts as such can be helpful in clinical decision-making, especially as such clusters of patients can be used to construct digital representations, or digital twins of the present patient to perform as clinical decision support tools (Wickramasinghe et al., 2024a, b).

Clustering Techniques

Numerous algorithms are available to perform clustering. In this section, some of the most common clustering algorithms that could be made use of with healthcare data are briefly described along with a clinical application scenario targeted at breast cancer.

K-Means Clustering

The K-Means algorithm (Na et al., 2010) can be used to divide a dataset into a "K"-number of distinct, non-overlapping clusters, or groups. The algorithm iteratively assigns each data point to the cluster that has the mean value nearest to the data point and thereby updates the cluster centroids until convergence. The process begins with the selection of K initial centroids at random. Each data point is then assigned to the nearest centroid based on Euclidean distance. The centroids are recalculated as the mean of all points in each cluster. This assignment and update process is repeated until the centroids stabilize.

In the context of breast cancer, K-Means can be used to segment patients into different categories based on their clinical and genetic data. Such a segmentation can help in identifying high-risk patients who may benefit from more aggressive screening and more personalized treatment plans, thereby providing clinical decision support.

Hierarchical Clustering

Hierarchical clustering (Murtagh & Contreras, 2017) can be used to build tree-like structures (or dendrograms) having nested clusters by either merging smaller clusters (agglomerative) or splitting larger clusters (divisive). The agglomerative approach starts with each data point as a single cluster and iteratively merges the closest pairs of clusters based on a chosen linkage criterion, such as single, complete, or average linkage. Conversely, the divisive approach begins with all data points in a single cluster and recursively splits them until each data point is in its own cluster.

In the context of cancer, hierarchical clustering can be used to create taxonomies to distinct tumour or patient subtypes, to help better understand the relationships between different tumour or patient characteristics and post-treatment outcomes. Such segmentations and entailing understanding can guide clinical decisions and the development of personalized treatment plans.

DBSCAN (Density-Based Spatial Clustering of Applications with Noise)

DBSCAN (Schubert et al., 2017) can be used to group data points that are densely or closely placed, and separate points in sparse regions as outliers. The algorithm requires two parameters: the first is the maximum distance between two points to be considered neighbours, and the second is the minimum number of points required to form a dense region. Core points are identified as those with at least neighbours within a boundary, and clusters are expanded from these core points to include all reachable points. Points not reachable from any core point are marked as outliers.

In the context of breast cancer, DBSCAN can be used to identify clusters of similar tumour or patient characteristics within large datasets. Such clustering can help detect rare subtypes of breast cancer that might be missed by other clustering methods or conventional screening and diagnosis. Such clustering can lead to more accurate diagnoses and the development of more personalized treatment strategies.

Gaussian Mixture Models (GMMs)

When using Gaussian mixture models (GMMs) (Reynolds, 2009), it is assumed that the data is generated from a mixture of several Gaussian distributions, each representing a different cluster. The Expectation-Maximization (EM) algorithm is used to estimate the parameters of these Gaussian distributions. First, the probability that each data point belongs to each Gaussian distribution is estimated. In the M-step, the parameters of the Gaussian distributions are updated to maximize the likelihood of the data. This process is repeated until the parameters converge.

In the context of breast cancer, GMMs can be used to model the distribution of tumour biomarkers or patient data and predict cancer progression and post-treatment outcomes. By probabilistically clustering such data, GMMs may be usable to identify patterns that can inform prognosis and treatment planning.

Mean-Shift Clustering

Mean-shift (Derpanis, 2005; Wu & Yang, 2007) is a non-parametric clustering technique that seeks to find the modes (or peaks) of a density function. The algorithm uses a bandwidth parameter to determine the size of the window used to compute the mean shift. For each data point, the mean of points within the bandwidth is computed, and the data point is shifted to this mean. This process is repeated until convergence to a mode.

In the context of breast cancer, mean-shift clustering can be used to segment tumours in mammograms, helping radiologists to accurately identify tumour boundaries and assess tumour shape and size, which are critical for diagnosis and treatment.

Affinity Propagation

Affinity propagation (Dueck, 2009) is a technique that can be used to identify representative points and thereby form clusters around such points based on passing messages between data points. A similarity matrix is constructed to measure the similarity between all pairs of data points. The algorithm iteratively updates two types of messages: responsibility, which measures how well suited a point is to be a representative point for another point, and availability, which measures how appropriate it is for a point to choose another point as its representative point. This process is continued until convergence is reached.

In the context of breast cancer, affinity propagation can be used to identify representative patients from large sets of past patient data. Such identification can help in capturing the diversity of patient profiles and responses to treatments. Such granular understanding can help the development of more personalized treatment plans.

Spectral Clustering

Spectral clustering (Jia et al., 2014) uses eigenvalues of a similarity matrix to perform dimensionality reduction before performing clustering based on fewer dimensions of data. The process involves constructing a similarity matrix representing the similarity between data points. This is followed by computing the graph Laplacian from this matrix, performing eigen decomposition on the Laplacian, and then applying a clustering algorithm like K-Means on the dataset that has been reduced in dimensionality.

In the context of breast cancer, spectral clustering can be used to analyse high-dimensional gene expression data, and sometimes spatial transcriptomics data, to identify clusters of genes in different tumour subtypes. Such clustering can provide insights about breast cancer tumour microenvironments, and thereby help identify potential targets for new therapies.

Self-Organizing Maps (SOMs)

Self-organizing maps (SOMs) (Kohonen, 2013) is a type of artificial neural network used to produce a low-dimensional (typically 2D) representation of high-dimensional data. The algorithm initializes the weight vectors of the neurons on a grid and, for each data point, finds the neuron with the closest weight vector (best matching unit). The weight vectors of the best matching unit and its neighbours are then updated to be closer to the data point. This process is repeated for a specified number of iterations.

In the context of breast cancer, SOMs can be used to visualize complex patient data, such as genetic profiles and spatial transcriptomics data, helping to identify patterns and correlations that may not be apparent to human observation of higher dimensional data. Such visualization aids help in understanding the heterogeneity of breast cancer and thereby help in developing more targeted and personalized treatment strategies.

Discussion

As discussed above, clustering algorithms can offer numerous strengths in healthcare applications. They can provide clinical decision support, and thereby help improve diagnostic and treatment accuracy by identifying patterns and anomalies in large datasets. This is particularly beneficial in managing chronic diseases like cancer. Breast cancer was discussed above as an example. Additionally, these algorithms enable the personalization of treatment plans by grouping patients and conditions with similar characteristics, thus tailoring treatments to individual needs. This is especially valuable in oncology, where treatment responses can vary widely among patients. Furthermore, clustering can streamline clinical workflows by auto-mating the sorting and categorization of patient data, reducing the workload on healthcare professionals and allowing them to focus more on providing care to the patients. These algorithms can also provide data-driven insights by uncovering hidden patterns and correlations, which can be invaluable for both research and clinical practice.

However, there are several weaknesses associated with clustering algo-rithms. Their effectiveness heavily depends on the quality and complete-ness of the data available for learning. Incomplete or noisy data can lead to inaccurate results. Some clustering techniques, such as GMMs and Spectral Clustering, can be complex and difficult to interpret, making it challenging for clinicians to understand and trust the results. Additionally, certain algo-rithms, like Hierarchical Clustering, may not scale well with very large data-sets, which are common in healthcare settings.

There are also significant opportunities to integrate clustering algorithms in healthcare. They can be integrated with Electronic Health Records (EHRs) to provide real-time decision support, enhancing the quality of care. These algorithms can also be used in predictive analytics to forecast the likes of disease progression (in the context of chronic diseases like cancer), patient readmissions, critical events, and side-effects, allowing for proactive health-care management. Clustering can also facilitate the development of personal-ized treatment by identifying patient subgroups that respond differently to treatments, leading to more effective and targeted therapies.

Despite aforesaid opportunities, there are also threats to the widespread adoption of clustering algorithms in healthcare. Privacy and security con-cerns are paramount, as the use of patient data for clustering raises significant issues. Ensuring data protection and compliance with local and international regulations is crucial. There may also be resistance to change among health-care professionals, especially if they perceive new technologies as complex or unreliable, or as a threat to their occupation. Ethical considerations must be carefully managed to avoid biases and ensure fair treatment of all patients and healthcare provider groups.

Several enablers can support the adoption of clustering algorithms in healthcare. Advancements in technology, such as improvements in computa-tional power and data storage capabilities, enable the efficient processing of large healthcare datasets. Supportive policies and regulations that promote the use of AI and ML in healthcare can facilitate the adoption of these tech-niques. Interdisciplinary collaboration between engineers, data scientists, cli-nicians, healthcare administrators, policy makers, ethicists, investors, and so on is essential for the next-generation leap in healthcare through AI and ML.

Barriers to the adoption of clustering algorithms and other ML techniques in healthcare are multi-faceted. These include challenges, such as the need for specialized knowledge and expertise, and the need for initial invest-ment in technology and training. Such challenges can be a barrier in some healthcare settings. Additionally, fragmented and siloed data systems can hinder the effective use of clustering and other ML algorithms in healthcare, as comprehensive and integrated datasets are essential for effective training of ML algorithms.

Conclusions

This chapter discussed the possibility of leveraging ML clustering techniques for enhanced clinical decision support within healthcare. It can be concluded that clustering algorithms hold significant promise for enhancing clinical decision support in healthcare. This can result in improving diagnostic accuracy, personalizing treatment plans, and streamlining clinical workflows. However, their successful implementation requires addressing challenges related to data quality, interpretability, scalability, privacy, and ethical considerations. With advancements in technology, supportive policies, and interdisciplinary collaboration, the barriers to adoption can be overcome with time and focused effort, paving the way for a more data-driven and personalized approach in healthcare. The potential for transformative impact of clustering techniques and ML and AI on clinical decision-making highlights the importance of continued research and development in this field.

References

Bijani, M., Abedi, S., Karimi, S., & Tehranineshat, B. (2021). Major challenges and barriers in clinical decision-making as perceived by emergency medical services personnel: A qualitative content analysis. *BMC Emergency Medicine, 21*(1), 12.

Derpanis, K. G. (2005). Mean shift clustering. *Lecture Notes, 32*(1–4), 16.

Dueck, D. (2009). *Affinity propagation: Clustering data by passing messages.* University of Toronto.

Jain, A. K. (2010). Data clustering: 50 years beyond K-means. *Pattern Recognition Letters, 31*(8), 651–666.

Jia, H., Ding, S., Xu, X., & Nie, R. (2014). The latest research progress on spectral clustering. *Neural Computing and Applications, 24*, 1477–1486.

Kohonen, T. (2013). Essentials of the self-organizing map. *Neural Networks, 37*, 52–65.

Krislock, N., & Wolkowicz, H. (2012). *Euclidean distance matrices and applications.* Springer.

Murtagh, F., & Contreras, P. (2017). Algorithms for hierarchical clustering: An overview, II. *Wiley Interdisciplinary Reviews: Data Mining and Knowledge Discovery, 7*(6), e1219.

Na, S., Xumin, L., & Yong, G. (2010). Research on k-means clustering algorithm: An improved k-means clustering algorithm. *2010 Third International Symposium on intelligent information technology and security informatics.* Jian, China, 63–67. https://doi.org/10.1109/IITSI.2010.74

Reynolds, D. A. (2009). Gaussian mixture models. *Encyclopedia of Biometrics, 741,* 659–663.

Schubert, E., Sander, J., Ester, M., Kriegel, H. P., & Xu, X. (2017). DBSCAN revisited, revisited: Why and how you should (still) use DBSCAN. *ACM Transactions on Database Systems (TODS), 42*(3), 1–21.

Watkins, S. (2020). Effective decision-making: Applying the theories to nursing practice. *British Journal of Nursing, 29*(2), 98–101.

Wickramasinghe, N., Ulapane, N., Sloane, E. B., & Gehlot, V. (2024a). Digital twins for more precise and personalized treatment. In *MEDINFO 2023—The future is accessible* (pp. 229–233). IOS Press.

Wickramasinghe, N., Ulapane, N., Zelcer, J., & Saffery, R. (2024b). 'Omics-based digital twins for personalised paediatric healthcare. *Studies in Health Technology and Informatics, 318,* 180–181.

Wu, K.-L., & Yang, M.-S. (2007). Mean shift-based clustering. *Pattern Recognition, 40*(11), 3035–3052.

Wu, X., Xiao, L., Sun, Y., Zhang, J., Ma, T., & He, L. (2022). A survey of human-in-the-loop for machine learning. *Future Generation Computer Systems, 135,* 364–381.

Ye, J. (2011). Cosine similarity measures for intuitionistic fuzzy sets and their applications. *Mathematical and Computer Modelling, 53*(1–2), 91–97.

5

Clinical Decision Support through Federated Learning and Blockchain

Introduction

Evolution of Healthcare and Clinical Decision-Making

The evolution of healthcare has been marked by significant advancements in technology and medical knowledge, leading to improved patient outcomes and more efficient healthcare delivery. Central to this evolution is clinical decision-making [1, 2], which has transitioned from being solely reliant on the expertise of healthcare professionals to incorporating sophisticated decision support systems [3]. These systems leverage vast amounts of health data and advanced analytics to provide evidence-based recommendations [4], thereby enhancing the accuracy and effectiveness of clinical decisions.

Challenges in Health Data Sharing for Intelligent Clinical Decision-Making

In today's healthcare landscape, the sharing of health data is crucial for intelligent clinical decision-making. Access to diverse and comprehensive datasets enables the development of robust machine learning models that can predict patient outcomes, identify potential health risks, and recommend personalized treatment plans [5]. However, this data sharing is fraught with challenges, including privacy concerns, regulatory constraints, and the risk of data breaches [6, 7]. These issues hinder the seamless exchange of health information, limiting the potential benefits of data-driven clinical decision support.

Importance of Federated Data and the Role of Federated Learning and Blockchain

One way of addressing the aforesaid challenges associated with health data sharing is by keeping health data federated, meaning that data remains within the custodianship of individual healthcare providers. This approach mitigates the risks associated with data sharing while still enabling collaborative learning. Federated learning (FL) [8], combined with blockchain technology [9, 10], offers a solution by allowing healthcare providers to share

DOI: 10.1201/9781003485971-7

machine learning models rather than raw data. This model-sharing approach ensures data privacy and security while facilitating the collective advancement of clinical decision support systems.

Advancements in Machine Learning and the Role of Federated Learning

Machine learning has revolutionized intelligent clinical decision-making by providing tools that can analyse complex health data and generate actionable insights [3]. FL [8] represents a significant evolution within this field, allowing models to be trained across multiple decentralized datasets without compromising data privacy. This decentralized approach aligns with the broader trend in machine learning towards more secure and collaborative methods.

Blockchain Technology and Its Application in Healthcare Model Sharing

The emergence of blockchain technology [9] has further transformed data sharing by providing a secure and transparent platform for exchanging information. In healthcare, in addition to raw data [10], blockchain can be utilized to share machine learning models, ensuring that sensitive health information remains protected. This technology enables the creation of a trusted network where healthcare providers can access and validate models from other institutions, enhancing the overall quality of clinical decision support.

Integrating Federated Learning and Blockchain to Address Healthcare Data Sharing Issues

This paper amalgamates FL and blockchain to address the issues associated with healthcare data sharing. By leveraging these technologies, we aim to answer the following research question: How might FL and blockchain be leveraged to ensure secure, efficient, and collaborative clinical decision support in healthcare? Through this exploration, we demonstrate the potential of these technologies to transform the landscape of clinical decision-making, particularly in the context of chronic disease management and cancer care.

Literature Review

Federated Learning in Healthcare

FL has emerged as a promising approach to address the challenges of data privacy and security in healthcare. By enabling the training of machine learning models across decentralized data sources without the need to share raw data, FL preserves patient privacy while leveraging the collective knowledge of multiple institutions. A review by Dhade and Shirke [11] highlights the potential of FL in healthcare, emphasizing its ability to enhance data-driven insights while maintaining data security. This review discusses various aspects of FL, including algorithmic aspects, privacy preservation, and several application contexts demonstrating the versatility and effectiveness of FL in different healthcare contexts.

Another systematic review by Prayitno et al. [12] explores the implementation of FL in healthcare from the perspective of data properties and applications. The authors identify key challenges such as data heterogeneity, communication and connectivity, model convergence, and more. They also highlight several healthcare case studies where FL has been applied, such as autism spectrum disorder, cancer diagnosis, COVID-19 detection, human activity and emotion recognition, patient hospitalization prediction, patient mortality prediction, and sepsis disease diagnosis.

Blockchain Technology in Healthcare

Blockchain technology offers a decentralized and transparent framework for secure data storage and sharing, making it an ideal solution for addressing the challenges of data integrity and privacy in healthcare. Khezr et al. [13] provide a review of blockchain applications in healthcare, outlining its potential to revolutionize data management and enhance the security of health data. The review discusses various use cases, including data management, supply chain management, and clinical trial management, highlighting the benefits of blockchain in ensuring data integrity and reducing fraud.

Agbo et al. [14] have conducted a systematic review, reporting on the ongoing research in the use of blockchain technology in healthcare. The authors have identified several barriers to implementation of blockchain in healthcare, such as lack of interoperability among disparate systems, lack of standards, lack of scalability, high volume of clinical data, lack of patient engagement and willingness to manage their own data, issues with data security and privacy, and lack of incentives for the uptake of blockchain technologies. The authors have also presented case studies demonstrating the successful and potential integration of blockchain in healthcare, such as in the management of electronic medical records, health supply chain management, biomedical research and education, elimination of falsification of data and the under-reporting or exclusion of undesirable results in clinical research, remote patient monitoring, health insurance claims, and health data analytics.

Such research hint that by integrating FL and blockchain technology, there is potential for the healthcare providers to create a secure and efficient framework for collaborative clinical decision-making. The works that were reviewed highlight this potential to transform healthcare by addressing the critical issues of data privacy, security, and interoperability.

Liquid Neural Networks (LNNs)

Later in this paper, we present a use case of how liquid neural networks (LNNs) can be used to build data-driven models to assist with clinical decision-making. Therefore, this subsection is dedicated to briefly review LNNs.

LNNs represent an innovative and rapidly developing area within machine learning. The review in this section draws on several key references [15–18] to provide an overview of LNNs.

The consensus among these studies is that LNNs possess a unique capability to adapt to temporal data. This adaptability stems from their design as systems of linear first-order dynamical systems, which are modulated by nonlinear interlinked gates [17]. This configuration allows LNNs to maintain stable and bounded behaviour, offering superior expressivity within the realm of neural ordinary differential equations, and enhancing performance in time-series prediction tasks [17].

A notable strength of LNNs is their ability to self-adapt to sudden changes in data patterns without the need for retraining [15]. This makes them particularly valuable for applications involving dynamic temporal data. Additionally, LNNs excel at learning and predicting gradients, or the rate of change in dynamic temporal data, which is beneficial for tasks such as traffic forecasting [15] and other time-series predictions [16, 17].

Beyond these applications, LNNs have been utilized in diverse fields such as robotics, causality analysis [16], and even in modelling liquid splash dynamics [18]. They are also being optimized for use in embedded systems that have limited computational resources and stringent performance requirements [16].

In this paper, we leverage the adaptability and gradient prediction capabilities of LNNs to explore their potential as digital twins for patients in healthcare. Specifically, we focus on forecasting patient progression in chronic diseases like cancer, thereby assessing the feasibility of using LNNs as tools for clinical decision support.

Methodology and Results

Clinical Scenario Performed by One Hospital (Denoted as Hospital A)

Suppose a hospital (denoted as Hospital A) receives an $N, N \in \mathbb{Z}^+$ number of patients who are diagnosed with a certain type of cancer. Each of these patients go through a certain number of clinical encounters equally spaced in time. At the mth clinical encounter ($m \in \mathbb{Z}^+$) the radius of a cancer tumour of the kth patient ($k \in \mathbb{Z}^+, k \le N$) remains $y_m^{(k)}$, $y_m^{(k)} \in \mathbb{R}^+$, $\forall m, k$ and the patient receives a clinical intervention (such as a dosage of chemotherapy) denoted as $x_m^{(k)}$, $x_m^{(k)} \in \mathbb{R}^+$, $0.1 \le x_m^{(k)} \le 0.9$, $\forall m, k$. It is assumed that the initial conditions remain $0.5 \le y_1^{(k)} \le 0.9$, $\forall k$ and $x_1^{(k)} = 0.5$, $\forall k$. At this stage suppose the clinicians have minimal facility for modeling, and therefore at the subsequent clinical encounters the intervention $x_m^{(k)}$, $m \geq 2$, is decided by the clinician to be a random number such that $0.1 \leq x_m^{(k)} \leq 0.9$, $\forall m, k$. For modeling purposes it is assumed that under the above condition the tumour radii of all patients vary according to equation (5.1) where $\epsilon_m^{(k)}$, $\epsilon_m^{(k)} \in \mathbb{R}$ is additive and random noise such that $|\epsilon_m^{(k)}| \leq 0.05 y_m^{(k)}$, $\forall m, k$, and the parameters $\alpha^{(k)}, \beta^{(k)}$ are such that $\alpha^{(k)} = 1$, $\forall k$, and $\beta^{(k)} \in \mathbb{R}^+$, $0.1 \leq \beta^{(k)} \leq 0.9$, $\beta^{(k)} \sim \mathcal{N}(0.5, 0.1^2)$, $\forall k$. In the clinical context, $\epsilon_m^{(k)}$ is not measurable by the clinician. The parameters $\alpha^{(k)}, \beta^{(k)}$ are not known to the clinician and are not measurable. The clinician only measures $y_m^{(k)}$ and prescribes $x_m^{(k)}$. Suppose hospital A receives $N = 385$ such patients and they are treated across $m = 1, 2, 3, \ldots, 5$ clinical encounters, and suppose this data is recorded.

$$y_{m+1}^{(k)} = \alpha^{(k)} y_m^{(k)} + \beta^{(k)} \left(x_m^{(k)} - 0.5 \right) + \epsilon_m^{(k)} \tag{5.1}$$

An Analytics Exploration Performed Hospital A

Now suppose an analytics exploration is done. An adapting neural network carrying one hidden layer with r, $r \in \mathbb{Z}^+$ number of neurons and one output layer is designed to take $2m$ inputs at the mth clinical encounter and model the tumor progression as in equation (5.3) using the commonly used hyperbolic tangent activation function $\tanh(t)$ for $t \in \mathbb{R}$ given in (2) [19]. As such, this neural network adapts according to the clinical encounter m, and outputs the tumor growth rate for patient k expected until the subsequent clinical encounter, thereby representing the attributes of a LNN in terms of adaptability and predicting rate of change [15, 16]. The model parameters $u_i^{(m)}, v_i^{(m)}, w_j^{(m)}, b_1^{(m)}, b_2^{(m)} \in \mathbb{R}$ are learned from the data of the $N = 385$ patients described earlier by splitting into training (50% of the data), testing (25%) and validation (25%) sets ensuring model reliability and overfit avoidance. The performance of the neural network for the 4rd clinical encounter, i.e., $m = 4$, is shown in Figure 5.1 as an example. After learning the parameters for each clinical encounter, suppose Hospital A publishes those parameters for the benefits of other hospitals through a means such as a dedicated healthcare blockchain.

$$\tanh(t) = \frac{e^t - e^{-t}}{e^t + e^{-t}} \tag{5.2}$$

$$\widehat{y_{m+1}^{(k)} - y_m^{(k)}} = \sum_{j=1}^{r} w_j^{(m)} \tanh\left(\sum_{i=1}^{m} u_i^{(m)} x_i^{(k)} + v_i^{(m)} y_i^{(k)} + b_1^{(m)} \right) + b_2^{(m)} \tag{5.3}$$

Hospital A's Models Being Used by Another Hospital (Hospital B)

Now suppose another hospital (Hospital B) receives another cohort of similar cancer patients governed by the same constraints described for Hospital A.

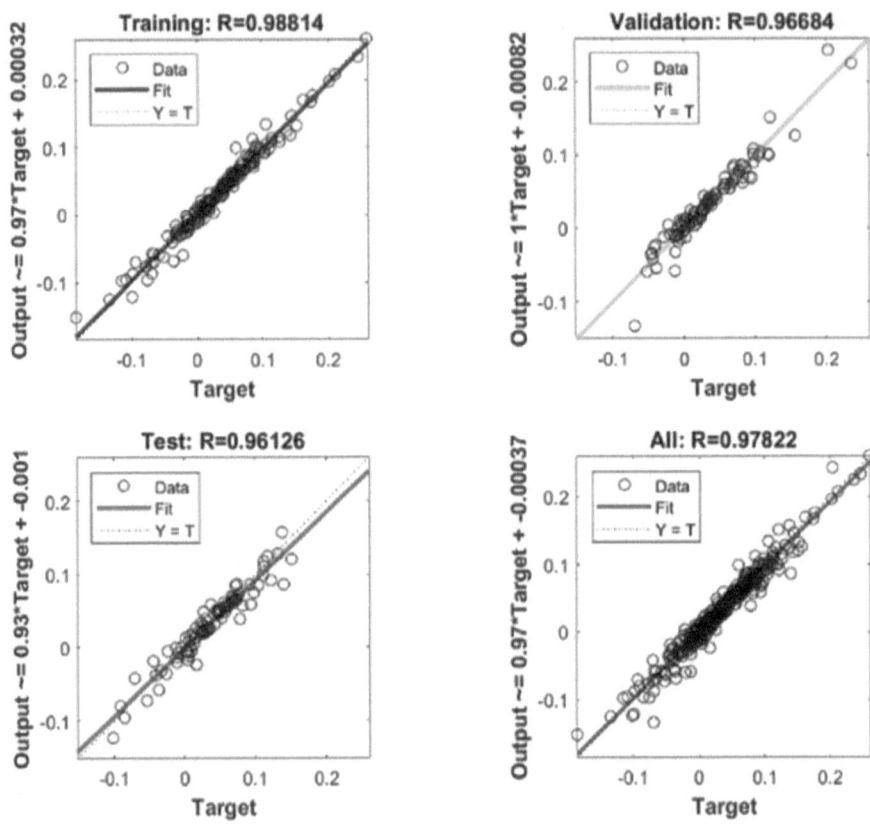

FIGURE 5.1
Performance example of a neural network; the one learned for clinical encounter 4.

Hospital B treats these patients with $x_1^{(k)} = 0.5$, $\forall k$ at the first clinical encounter. However, in the subsequent clinical encounters, the treatment intensity is calculated by solving the minimization problem shown in equation (5.4), where the objective is to reduce the tumour radii to some desired threshold denoted by y_{ref}, $y_{ref} \in \mathbb{R}^+$. For computation purposes, we set $y_{ref} = 0.1$. The notation $\|\dashv\|$ indicates the Euclidian norm. As such, Hospital B derives some intelligent decision support through the models generated by Hospital A. The outcomes of this clinical intervention assisted by intelligent clinical decision support are shown in Figures 5.2 and 5.3. As shown in those figures, a significant improvement in clinical outcomes can be seen through this numerical example, demonstrating the feasibility and the likely impact of the proposed approach.

$$x_m^{(k)*} = \arg\min_{x_m^{(k)}} \left\| \widehat{y}_{m+1}^{(k)} - y_{ref} \right\|^2 \tag{5.4}$$

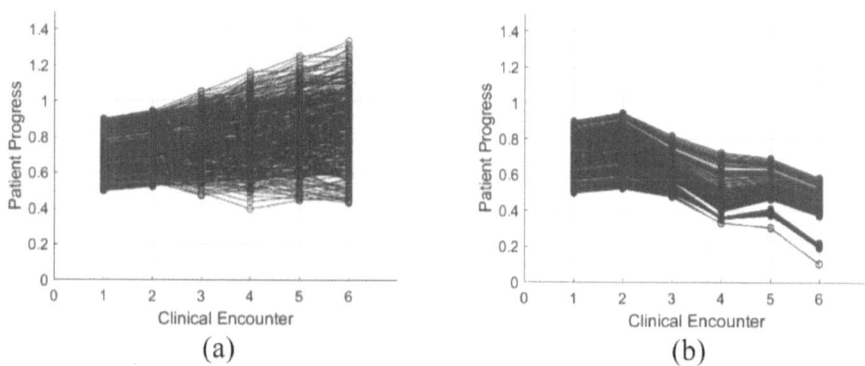

FIGURE 5.2

Tumour progression (i.e., variation of tumour radii): (a) 385 patients from Hospital A that underwent the standard treatment protocol; (b) 385 patients from Hospital B that underwent treatment assisted by intelligent decision support derived through LNN models produced by Hospital A.

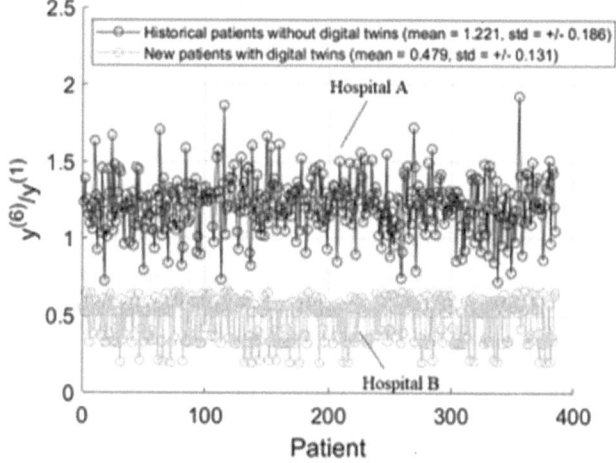

FIGURE 5.3

Impact of model sharing and intelligent clinical decision support: relative reduction of tumour size, i.e., $y_6^{(k)}/y_1^{(k)}$.

Discussion

Summary of the Conducted Work

This paper presented a numerical example using synthetic data to demonstrate the application of LNNs in modelling cancer tumour radius. This paper showed how LNNs can be utilized for treatment planning and clinical decision support. This paper further showed the process by which one hospital can develop such models using its own data and share these models, rather than the data itself, with other healthcare providers via blockchain technology. This paper also demonstrated how another hospital could leverage these shared models for its own clinical decision support, ultimately improving patient outcomes. This paper highlighted the feasibility of using FL and model sharing, facilitated by blockchain, as an alternative to data sharing in healthcare.

Contribution to Theory

Exemplifying the Use of LNNs in a Healthcare Setting

This paper contributes to the theoretical understanding of LNNs by exemplifying their application in a healthcare setting. By modelling cancer tumour radius, the paper highlights the potential of LNNs to support clinical decision-making processes. The use of LNNs in this context demonstrates their capability to handle dynamic data, providing a robust tool for treatment planning and enhancing the precision of clinical decisions. Extending further, the proposed LNN models when being used for clinical decision support for a particular patient, can be interpreted as a digital twin of that particular patient.

Exemplifying the Impact of Model Sharing in a Healthcare Setting

This paper also contributes to theory by illustrating the impact of model sharing in healthcare. By enabling hospitals to share learned models instead of raw data, this paper addresses significant privacy and security concerns associated with health data sharing. This approach not only facilitates collaborative learning and improvement of clinical decision support systems but also ensures that sensitive patient data remains protected.

Contribution to Practice

An Approach to Use Blockchain to Share Models Instead of Data in a Healthcare Setting

From a practical standpoint, this paper proposed an approach to use blockchain technology for sharing machine learning models in healthcare. By leveraging blockchain, hospitals can securely share models, ensuring transparency and traceability while maintaining data privacy. This method allows healthcare providers to benefit from advanced clinical decision support tools without the risks associated with data sharing, thereby enhancing patient care and operational efficiency whilst preserving data privacy and security.

Limitations of This Study

A Numerical Example

One limitation of this paper is the work being based on numerical examples based on synthetic data, simulating the interplay between two hospitals.

While the results are promising, it must be noted that real-world applications may present additional challenges that must be learned through real-world data. Future studies should consider more extensive datasets and involve multiple healthcare providers to build on the prospective findings of this paper and ensure the development of scalable and robust solutions.

Conclusions and Future Work

This chapter demonstrates the feasibility and benefits of using LNNs through FL for clinical decision support and the potential of blockchain-facilitated model sharing in healthcare. The findings suggest that FL and model sharing can address intelligent data-driven clinical decision support whilst preserving data privacy and addressing data security issues inherent in health data sharing.

Future work will focus on expanding further to include more hospitals and real-world data, exploring the integration of other advanced machine learning models, and further investigating the long-term impacts on patient outcomes and healthcare operations. Additionally, addressing specific concerns related to health data sharing, such as data ownership, consent, and regulatory compliance, will be crucial for the broader adoption of approaches such as the one presented in the preceding section.

Acknowledgement

OPTUS and La Trobe University, Australia are acknowledged for their support for this research.

References

1. M. Banning, "A review of clinical decision making: Models and current research," *Journal of Clinical Nursing*, vol. 17, no. 2, pp. 187–195, 2008.
2. N. Ulapane, and N. Wickramasinghe, "Clinical Decision-Making as a Subset of Decision-Making: Leveraging the Concepts of Decision-Making and Knowledge Management to Characterize Clinical Decision-Making," in *Healthcare and Knowledge Management for Society 5.0*, 2021: CRC Press, pp. 47–62.
3. A. E. Andargoli, N. Ulapane, T. A. Nguyen, N. Shuakat, J. Zelcer, and N. Wickramasinghe, "Intelligent decision support systems for dementia care: A scoping review," *Artificial Intelligence in Medicine*, p. 102815, 2024. https://doi.org/10.1016/j.artmed.2024.102815

4. M. A. Musen, B. Middleton, and R. A. Greenes, "Clinical Decision-Support Systems," in *Biomedical Informatics: Computer Applications in Health Care and Biomedicine*, 2021: Springer, pp. 795–840.

5. I. Bica, A. M. Alaa, C. Lambert, and M. Van Der Schaar, "From real-world patient data to individualized treatment effects using machine learning: Current and future methods to address underlying challenges," *Clinical Pharmacology & Therapeutics*, vol. 109, no. 1, pp. 87–100, 2021.

6. J. P. Hlávka, "Security, Privacy, and Information-Sharing Aspects of Healthcare Artificial Intelligence," in *Artificial Intelligence in Healthcare*, 2020: Elsevier, pp. 235–270.

7. N. Ulapane, and N. Wickramasinghe, "Critical Issues in Mobile Solution-Based Clinical Decision Support Systems: A Scoping Review," in *Optimizing Health Monitoring Systems with Wireless Technology*, N. Wickramasinghe Ed. 2021: IGI Global, pp. 32–45.

8. L. Li, Y. Fan, M. Tse, and K.-Y. Lin, "A review of applications in federated learning," *Computers & Industrial Engineering*, vol. 149, p. 106854, 2020.

9. A. G. Gad, D. T. Mosa, L. Abualigah, and A. A. Abohany, "Emerging trends in blockchain technology and applications: A review and outlook," *Journal of King Saud University-Computer and Information Sciences*, vol. 34, no. 9, pp. 6719–6742, 2022.

10. N. Ulapane, A. Eslami Andargoli, J. Miltner, J. van de Logt, M. Kraus, and F. Bodendorf, "A Suggested Blockchain Architecture for Healthcare Data Sharing," *AMCIS 2023 Proceedings*, 2023.

11. P. Dhade, and P. Shirke, "Federated learning for healthcare: A comprehensive review," *Engineering Proceedings*, vol. 59, no. 1, p. 230, 2024.

12. Prayitno, Shyu C-R, Putra KT, Chen H-C, Tsai Y-Y, Hossain KSMT, Jiang W, Shae Z-Y, "A systematic review of federated learning in the healthcare area: From the perspective of data properties and applications," *Applied Sciences*, vol. 11, no. 23, p. 11191, 2021. https://doi.org/10.3390/app112311191

13. S. Khezr, M. Moniruzzaman, A. Yassine, and R. Benlamri, "Blockchain technology in healthcare: A comprehensive review and directions for future research," *Applied Sciences*, vol. 9, no. 9, p. 1736, 2019.

14. C. C. Agbo, Q. H. Mahmoud, and J. M. Eklund, "Blockchain technology in healthcare: A systematic review," *Healthcare*, vol. 7, no. 2, p. 56, 2019.

15. O. Ayoub et al., "Liquid Neural Network-based Adaptive Learning vs. Incremental Learning for Link Load Prediction amid Concept Drift due to Network Failures," *arXiv preprint arXiv:2404.05304*, 2024.

16. M. Bidollahkhani, F. Atasoy, and H. Abdellatef, "LTC-SE: expanding the potential of liquid time-constant neural networks for scalable AI and embedded systems," *arXiv preprint arXiv:2304.08691*, 2023.

17. R. Hasani, M. Lechner, A. Amini, D. Rus, and R. Grosu, "Liquid time-constant networks," *Proceedings of the AAAI Conference on Artificial Intelligence*, vol. 35, no. 9, pp. 7657–7666, 2021.

18. K. Um, X. Hu, and N. Thuerey, "Liquid splash modeling with neural networks," *Computer Graphics Forum*, vol. 37, no. 8, 2018: Wiley Online Library, pp. 171–182.

19. S. K. Roy, S. Manna, S. R. Dubey, and B. B. Chaudhuri, "LiSHT: Non-parametric linearly scaled hyperbolic tangent activation function for neural networks," in *International Conference on Computer Vision and Image Processing*, 2022: Springer, pp. 462–476.

6

From Algorithms to Outcomes: Leveraging Machine Learning Classification Techniques for Enhanced Clinical Decision Support

Introduction

Clinical decision-making is a fundamental component of healthcare. It involves healthcare professionals assessing data about patients to make informed diagnoses and treatment choices. Accuracy in clinical decision-making is crucial for optimal patient outcomes and effective healthcare delivery. However, clinical decision-making encounters several challenges. Cognitive biases, for instance, is one challenge. It can lead to errors in judgements made by clinicians. This becomes so because clinicians may rely on heuristics that do not always align with evidence-based practices. Information overload is another challenge. This challenge arises because of the sheer volume of data that must be analysed by clinicians. Analysing vast amounts of data can overwhelm clinicians. This makes it difficult to discern relevant information quickly. Additionally, variability in the expertise of clinicians can also become a challenge. It results in inconsistent decision-making. That too further complicates patient care and potentially leads to suboptimal outcomes. Issues encountered in clinical decision-making are thus multifaceted (Bijani et al., 2021; Watkins, 2020). These issues highlight the need for enhanced decision support for clinicians. Enhanced clinical decision support can assist clinicians to navigate complex clinical scenarios.

Machine learning (ML) is a subset of artificial intelligence (AI). It has emerged as a promising solution that can address some of the above-mentioned challenges encountered in clinical decision-making. Through ML, algorithms can be designed and used to analyse vast and complex datasets. Through such analysis, complex patterns may be identified. These patterns may not be apparent to human clinicians. But through algorithms, such patterns can be discovered through computation. This capability allows for more informed decision-making. ML techniques can process information at a scale and speed that far exceeds human capacity (Wu et al., 2022).

Classification techniques play a significant role in ML. Classification allows categorizing data into predefined classes or labels (Kesavaraj & Sukumaran, 2013). In the context of healthcare and clinical decision-making, classification can help in tasks such as providing disease diagnosis assistance, predicting patient outcomes, and recommending treatments and treatment plans personalized based on health and medical data of patients. Employing classification techniques thus has the potential to enhance the likes of diagnostic accuracy and the personalization of treatment plans and clinical workflows.

This chapter explores various classification techniques. These techniques are explored particularly regarding their potential as clinical decision support tools. We look at how these techniques can be leveraged to support healthcare practices. Means such as improving diagnostic accuracy, personalizing treatment plans, and streamlining clinical workflows are particularly focused on. Furthermore, opportunities and barriers associated with the implementation of ML techniques in clinical settings are identified and briefly discussed. Thereby we attempt to highlight the transformative impact ML techniques can have on clinical decision-making by answering the research question: How might classification techniques enhance clinical decision support?

Classification: An Overview

In ML, classification is a supervised learning technique used to categorize data into predefined classes or labels. The process involves training a model on a labelled dataset, where the input data is paired with the correct output labels. In healthcare, as an example, a classification model could process different data elements of cancer patients and predict which treatment option the patient is likely to benefit from most. Here, the patient's data will be the input to a classifier. The output labels will be the treatment options available. A classifier model thus learns to identify patterns and relationships within the data, enabling it to predict the class of new, unseen instances. Common algorithms such as decision trees, support vector machines, and neural networks are used for classification (Boateng et al., 2020). The goal is to achieve high accuracy in predicting the correct class for each input, making classification a fundamental task useful for many applications including performing as clinical decision support systems (CDSSs) in healthcare.

In the healthcare context, classification can be performed as follows. First, relevant data must be collected. This means, relevant data such as data of patients, such as medical history, laboratory results, and imaging, must be collected. Next, data preprocessing must be performed. This means, the data must be cleaned and prepared for analysis. This includes handling missing values, normalizing data, encoding categorical variables, and so on. Next, feature selection must be done. This means, relevant features (variables) that are most discriminative between classes should be selected to improve a classifier's performance. Various techniques such as statistical tests, correlation-based methods, recursive feature selection, regularization, principal component analysis, and so on are available for this (Cai et al., 2018). Next, a classifier model must be trained. Various ML algorithms, such as decision trees, support vector machines, or neural networks, are available for this (Boateng et al., 2020). These can be trained on the pre-processed data to learn patterns and relationships. Through these classifiers, classification happens. This means, the trained models are used to classify new data. In the healthcare context, this could mean certain aspects or data about patients are used for classification. This data is mapped into categories, or classes, such as diagnosing a specific disease (i.e., positive or negative – two classes) or predicting the likelihood of a certain prognosis, for example, the likelihood of success of a particular treatment given for a certain type of cancer of a certain patient. These classifier models must then be rigorously evaluated. This means the performance of these classifier models must be evaluated using metrics such as accuracy, precision, recall, and F1-score to ensure the classifiers provide reliable predictions (Hicks et al., 2022).

For example, certain CDSSs might benefit from using classification techniques to identify whether a patient has a high risk of a certain disease, heart disease for instance (Olsen et al., 2020), based on their medical history and current health-related data. This helps clinicians make informed decisions and provide timely interventions.

The key advantage in such ML techniques is that they can process large volumes of data faster than a human whilst being true to some statistical criteria and defined algorithms (Zhou et al., 2017). They can thus be used to assist as decision support tools. In healthcare, this means they can be helpful as clinical decision support tools.

Classification Techniques

Numerous algorithms are available to perform classification. In this section, some of the most common classification algorithms that could be made use of within the healthcare sector are briefly described along with a clinical application scenario targeted at breast cancer.

Logistic Regression

Logistic regression (Hosmer Jr et al., 2013) is a linear model used for binary classification tasks. It estimates the probability that a given input belongs to a particular class. The model uses the logistic function (sigmoid function) to map predicted values to probabilities between 0 and 1. The decision boundary is determined by a threshold, typically 0.5.

In the context of breast cancer, logistic regression can be used to predict the probability of a breast tumour being malignant based on features like tumour size, shape, and texture. This helps in improving diagnostic accuracy through clinical decision support.

Decision Trees

Decision trees (De Ville, 2013) are non-linear models that split the data into subsets based on the value of input features. Each internal node represents a feature, each branch represents a decision rule, and each leaf node represents an outcome. The tree is built using algorithms like ID3, C4.5, or classification and regression trees (CART), which select the best feature to split the data based on criteria like Gini impurity or information gain (Singh & Gupta, 2014).

In a clinical context, decision trees can be used to predict the best treatment options for breast cancer patients by analysing patient data such as age, tumour stage, and genetic markers. This helps in personalizing treatment plans and improving outcomes.

Support Vector Machines (SVM)

Support vector machines (SVMs) (Chandra & Bedi, 2021) are powerful classifiers that find the optimal hyperplane that maximizes the margin between different classes. For non-linear data, SVMs use kernel functions (e.g., polynomial, radial basis function) to transform the data into a higher-dimensional space where a linear separator can be found.

Regarding breast cancer, SVMs can classify breast cancer images from mammograms, distinguishing between normal and abnormal tissues (Chandra & Bedi, 2021). This aids radiologists in early detection and diagnosis.

K-Nearest Neighbours (KNN)

K-Nearest Neighbours (KNN) (Wang et al., 2022) is a simple, instance-based learning algorithm that classifies data points based on the majority class of their (k) nearest neighbours in the feature space. A distance metric (e.g., Euclidean distance) is used to find the nearest neighbours.

If applied in breast cancer, KNN can predict the likelihood of breast cancer recurrence by comparing a patient's data with similar past cases. This helps in predicting the likelihood of readmission and planning follow-up care.

Random Forest

Random Forest (Palimkar et al., 2022) is an ensemble method that builds multiple decision trees and merges their results to improve accuracy and control overfitting. Each tree is trained on a random subset of the data and features, and the final prediction is made by averaging the predictions of all trees (for regression) or taking a majority vote (for classification).

In breast cancer, the Random Forest method can be used to predict the success of different breast cancer treatment options by analysing a large dataset of patient outcomes. This helps in identifying the most effective treatment options for new patients.

Naive Bayes

Naive Bayes classifiers (Peretz et al., 2024) apply Bayes' theorem with the assumption of independence between features. It calculates the posterior probability of each class given the input features and selects the class with the highest probability.

In breast cancer, the Naive Bayes method can classify breast cancer patients into different risk categories based on genetic and lifestyle factors. This helps in early intervention and preventive care.

Neural Networks

Neural networks consist of interconnected layers of nodes (neurons) that process input data and learn complex patterns through backpropagation. Each neuron applies a weighted sum of inputs, passes it through an activation function, and propagates the result to the next layer. This approach can be programmed to ultimately match inputs to different output classes, sometimes through incorporating deep learning also (Shajin et al., 2023).

Relating to breast cancer, neural networks can analyse histopathology images to detect breast cancer cells with high accuracy. This supports pathologists in making precise diagnoses and treatment decisions.

Discussion

As discussed above, classification algorithms can offer numerous strengths and benefits through various applications in the healthcare sector. They can provide clinical decision support and thereby help improve diagnostic and treatment accuracy by mapping different data elements into predefined classes or groups. This is particularly beneficial as diagnostic and treatment planning clinical decision support tools, especially relating to chronic diseases like cancer. Breast cancer was discussed above as an example in this chapter. Additionally, these algorithms enable the personalization of treatment plans by grouping patients and conditions with similar characteristics, thus tailoring treatments to individual needs. This is especially valuable in chronic and complex scenarios like oncology, where treatment responses can vary widely among patients. Furthermore, classification can streamline clinical workflows by helping automation through categorization of different elements of data such as patient data and reducing the workload on health-care professionals and allowing them to focus more on providing care to the patients. These algorithms can also provide data-driven insights by uncovering hidden patterns and correlations through processing large volumes of data in short spans of time, and this can be invaluable for both research and clinical practice.

However, there are several weaknesses associated with classification algorithms. Their effectiveness heavily depends on the quality and completeness of the data available for learning. Incomplete or noisy data can lead to inaccurate results. Some classification techniques can be complex and difficult to interpret alongside taking longer times and higher power for computation, making it challenging for clinicians and hospitals to implement them in practice and use them. Such algorithms can also be difficult to understand inhibiting their interpretability and explainability, and this may reduce the trust the clinicians will have in the results. Additionally, certain algorithms may not scale well with very large datasets, which are common in health-care settings.

There are also significant opportunities to integrate classification algorithms in healthcare. They can be integrated with Electronic Health Records (EHRs) to provide real-time decision support, enhancing the quality of care. These algorithms can also be used in predictive analytics in tasks like disease diagnosis, treatment planning, patient readmissions, critical events, and side-effects, allowing for proactive healthcare management. Classification can also facilitate the development of personalized treatment by identifying which treatment options are most likely to be beneficial for a particular patient.

Despite aforesaid opportunities, there are also threats to the widespread adoption of classification algorithms in healthcare. Privacy and security concerns are paramount, as the use of patient data for classification raises significant issues. Ensuring data protection and compliance with local and international regulations is crucial. There may also be resistance to change among healthcare professionals, especially if they perceive new technologies as complex or unreliable, or as a threat to their occupation. Ethical considerations must also be carefully managed to avoid biases and ensure fair treatment to all patients and healthcare professionals and provider groups.

Several enablers can support the adoption of classification algorithms in healthcare. Advancements in technology, such as improvements in computational power and data storage capabilities, enable the efficient processing of large healthcare datasets. Supportive policies and regulations that promote the use of AI and ML in healthcare can facilitate the adoption of these techniques. Interdisciplinary collaboration between engineers, data scientists, clinicians, healthcare administrators, policymakers, ethicists, investors, and so on is essential for the next-generation leap in healthcare through AI and ML (Wickramasinghe et al., 2021).

Barriers to the adoption of classification algorithms and other AI and ML techniques in healthcare are multifaceted. These include challenges, such as the need for specialized knowledge and expertise, and the need for initial investment in technology and training. Such challenges can be a barrier in some healthcare settings. Additionally, fragmented and siloed data systems can hinder the effective use of classification and other ML algorithms in healthcare, as comprehensive and integrated datasets are essential for effective training of ML algorithms.

Conclusions

This chapter discussed the possibility of leveraging ML-based classification techniques for enhanced clinical decision support within healthcare. It can be concluded that classification algorithms hold significant promise for enhancing clinical decision support in healthcare. This can result in improving diagnostic accuracy, personalizing treatment plans, and streamlining clinical workflows. However, their successful implementation requires addressing challenges related to data quality, interoperability, scalability, privacy, and ethical considerations. With advancements in technology, supportive policies, and interdisciplinary collaboration, the barriers to adoption can be overcome with time and focused effort, paving the way for a more data-driven and personalized approach in healthcare. The potential for transformative impact of classification techniques and ML and AI on clinical decision-making highlights the importance of continued research and development in this field.

References

Bijani, M., Abedi, S., Karimi, S., & Tehranineshat, B. (2021). Major challenges and barriers in clinical decision-making as perceived by emergency medical services personnel: A qualitative content analysis. *BMC Emergency Medicine, 21*(1), 12.

Boateng, E. Y., Otoo, J., & Abaye, D. A. (2020). Basic tenets of classification algorithms K-nearest-neighbor, support vector machine, random forest and neural network: A review. *Journal of Data Analysis and Information Processing, 8*(4), 341–357.

Cai, J., Luo, J., Wang, S., & Yang, S. (2018). Feature selection in machine learning: A new perspective. *Neurocomputing, 300*, 70–79.

Chandra, M. A., & Bedi, S. (2021). Survey on SVM and their application in image classification. *International Journal of Information Technology, 13*(5), 1–11.

De Ville, B. (2013). Decision trees. *Wiley Interdisciplinary Reviews: Computational Statistics, 5*(6), 448–455.

Hicks, S. A., Strümke, I., Thambawita, V., Hammou, M., Riegler, M. A., Halvorsen, P., & Parasa, S. (2022). On evaluation metrics for medical applications of artificial intelligence. *Scientific Reports, 12*(1), 5979.

Hosmer, D. W. Jr, Lemeshow, S., & Sturdivant, R. X. (2013). *Applied logistic regression.* John Wiley & Sons.

Kesavaraj, G., & Sukumaran, S. (2013). A study on classification techniques in data mining. *2013 fourth international conference on computing, communications and networking technologies (ICCCNT), IEEE,* 1–7.

Olsen, C. R., Mentz, R. J., Anstrom, K. J., Page, D., & Patel, P. A. (2020). Clinical applications of machine learning in the diagnosis, classification, and prediction of heart failure. *American Heart Journal, 229,* 1–17.

Palimkar, P., Shaw, R. N., & Ghosh, A. (2022). Machine learning technique to prognosis diabetes disease: Random forest classifier approach. *Advanced computing and intelligent technologies: proceedings of ICACIT 2021,* 219–244.

Peretz, O., Koren, M., & Koren, O. (2024). Naive Bayes classifier – An ensemble procedure for recall and precision enrichment. *Engineering Applications of Artificial Intelligence, 136,* 108972.

Shajin, F. H. P. S., Rajesh, P., & Nagoji Rao, V. K. (2023). Efficient framework for brain tumour classification using hierarchical deep learning neural network classifier. *Computer Methods in Biomechanics and Biomedical Engineering: Imaging & Visualization, 11*(3), 750–757.

Singh, S., & Gupta, P. (2014). Comparative study ID3, cart and C4. 5 decision tree algorithm: A survey. *International Journal of Advanced Information Science and Technology (IJAIST), 27*(27), 97–103.

Wang, Y., Pan, Z., & Dong, J. (2022). A new two-layer nearest neighbor selection method for kNN classifier. *Knowledge-Based Systems, 235,* 107604.

Watkins, S. (2020). Effective decision-making: Applying the theories to nursing practice. *British Journal of Nursing, 29*(2), 98–101.

Wickramasinghe, N., Jayaraman, P. P., Forkan, A. R. M., Ulapane, N., Kaul, R., Vaughan, S., & Zelcer, J. (2021). A vision for leveraging the concept of digital twins to support the provision of personalized cancer care. *IEEE Internet Computing, 26*(5), 17–24.

Wu, X., Xiao, L., Sun, Y., Zhang, J., Ma, T., & He, L. (2022). A survey of human-in-the-loop for machine learning. *Future Generation Computer Systems, 135,* 364–381.

Zhou, L., Pan, S., Wang, J., & Vasilakos, A. V. (2017). Machine learning on big data: Opportunities and challenges. *Neurocomputing, 237,* 350–361.

7

From Perceptron to Liquid Neural Networks: The Evolution of Neural Networks and Their Role in Black Box Modelling for Digital Twins in Healthcare

What Are Digital Twins?

A digital twin is a dynamic, digital representation of a physical entity. It integrates data from various sources, including sensors, Internet of Things (IoT) devices, and historical records, to create a comprehensive model that mirrors the physical object or system. This model can be used for simulation, testing, monitoring, and maintenance, providing valuable insights into performance and potential issues (Marr, 2022; Siemens, 2025; Walker, 2023; Zorchenko et al., 2024).

Key Elements and Characteristics of Digital Twins

Key Elements and Characteristics of Digital Twins Are Summarized in This Section

Real-Time Data Collection and Connectivity: Sensors and IoT devices collect data such as temperature, pressure, and performance metrics and more. Continuous communication between the physical entity and the digital twin ensures the virtual model remains accurate and up to date.

Integration of Analytics and AI Models

Algorithms are used to analyse the incoming data to identify trends, predict failures, and simulate scenarios, and so on.

Interactive Dashboards

User-friendly interfaces are typically provided to present complex data in a clear, actionable format.

DOI: 10.1201/9781003485971-9

Some Recent Industrial Applications of Digital Twins

The capabilities of digital twins are useful in various industries. Some real-world applications of digital twins as evidenced to date are discussed in this section.

Energy

General Electric (GE) has pioneered the implementation of high-precision digital twins for power plants and energy systems (Zorchenko et al., 2024), leveraging its extensive experience in this field. GE's approach to creating digital twins involves a combination of physical laws, engineering design expertise, and advanced measurement and control methods. Central to this process are artificial intelligence technologies, including pattern recognition, unstructured (multimodal) data analysis, and expert networks, which enhance the accuracy and functionality of the digital twins. A key component of GE's digital twin technology is the Predix simulation platform. Developed specifically for industrial Internet applications, Predix enables real-time analytical processing of vast amounts of machine data. This platform integrates sensor technologies and AI to provide comprehensive insights and predictive analytics, optimizing the performance and maintenance of power plants and energy systems. The capabilities and specifications of Predix highlight its role in transforming data into actionable intelligence, ensuring efficient and reliable operations. GE's digital twins exemplify the convergence of traditional engineering principles with cutting-edge AI and IoT technologies, setting a benchmark for innovation in the energy sector.

The Siemens Electrical Digital Twin (Siemens, 2025) is a cutting-edge solution designed to revolutionize the management of power grids. As part of the Siemens Xcelerator portfolio, this digital twin offers a digitalized model of the physical world, enabling utilities to plan, operate, and maintain their grids with unprecedented precision. In an era marked by decentralization and the rise of renewable energy sources, managing and exchanging complex data has become increasingly challenging. The Siemens Electrical Digital Twin is designed to address this by integrating vast amounts of digital data, ensuring that even the smallest details are accurately represented. This integration helps utilities avoid costly mistakes and prepares them for a sustainable digital future. A prime example of its application is at American Electric Power (AEP), the largest transmission grid operator in the US AEP is leveraging the Siemens Electrical Digital Twin to create a unified network model, breaking down data silos and enabling reliable planning, operation, and protection of their power grid. This implementation is a significant step towards accelerating digital transformation and ensuring the resilience of the power infrastructure. By choosing the Siemens Electrical Digital Twin, utilities can seamlessly weave their digital data together, paving the way for a more efficient and sustainable energy landscape.

Smart Cities

The world's first digital twin of a nation, Virtual Singapore (Walker, 2023), has shown promise in revolutionizing urban planning and management. Initiated by the Singapore Land Authority (SLA), this ambitious project involved aircraft equipped with laser scanners patrolling the skies to create a detailed digital copy of one of the most densely populated islands in the world. This initiative began in response to a series of damaging floods in 2011, highlighting the need for better land use and flood risk management.

Starting in 2012, the SLA embarked on creating a 3D map of Singapore. GPS Lands Singapore later collaborated with the SLA to develop Virtual Singapore using software from Bentley Systems. Laser-scanning aircraft and vehicles collected terrain and surface data, which was then integrated into a single platform. This platform allows users to view and verify information, aiding in urban planning and design.

Virtual Singapore provides a highly detailed 3D representation of the entire country, shared across various government agencies for asset management and decision-making. The project also includes a national subsurface digital twin, capturing underground utility assets to optimize land use and reduce risks during construction.

The digital twin helps manage land more efficiently, minimizes disruption to services, and enhances safety during engineering works. It also supports emergency services with disaster planning and simulates evacuation scenarios. Additionally, with the map, transport flows and pedestrian movements can be analysed to prevent bottlenecks.

Virtual Singapore's open and collaborative nature makes it accessible to the public, private, government, and research sectors. This fosters innovation and integration in smart city development, ensuring that urban planning lessons are learned and shared. As digital twin technology continues to evolve, its potential to transform cities and infrastructure becomes increasingly apparent, offering significant benefits in efficiency, safety, and sustainability.

Automotive Industry

Tesla's innovative use of digital twins involves creating a digital simulation of each of its cars (Marr, 2022). This simulation is built using data collected from sensors on the vehicles, which is then uploaded to the cloud. By leveraging this data, Tesla's AI algorithms can predict where faults and breakdowns are most likely to occur. This proactive approach minimizes the need for owners to take their cars to servicing stations for repairs and maintenance, significantly reducing the cost to the company for servicing cars under warranty. Additionally, it enhances the user experience by providing more reliable and hassle-free vehicle ownership. This leads to more satisfied customers and increases the likelihood of repeat business for Tesla. Overall, Tesla's digital twin technology not only optimizes maintenance and repair processes but also targeted at strengthening customer loyalty and satisfaction.

Benefits of Digital Twins

Several benefits of using digital twins can be identified and several key benefits are summarized in this section.

The ability to Perform Predictive Maintenance: By analysing real-time data, digital twins can help with predicting when maintenance is needed, reducing downtime and extending the lifespan of equipment (Marr, 2022; Walker, 2023).

Improved Efficiency: Digital twins enable the optimization of processes and systems, leading to increased efficiency and reduced costs (Marr, 2022; Siemens, 2025; Walker, 2023; Zorchenko et al., 2024).

Enhanced Decision-Making: Real-time insights and simulations allow for better-informed decisions, improving overall performance and outcomes (Walker, 2023).

Risk Mitigation: Simulating different scenarios helps identify potential risks and develop strategies to mitigate them (Siemens, 2025; Walker, 2023; Zorchenko et al., 2024).

Digital Twins in Healthcare

Several scenarios where the concept of digital twins has been applied in healthcare have been discussed in relation to genomics (Björnsson et al., 2020; Wickramasinghe et al., 2024), aged care (Liu et al., 2019), chronic diseases (Wickramasinghe et al., 2021, 2022), and clinical workflows (Wickramasinghe et al., 2023), mostly targeted at improving precision and personalization of care (Björnsson et al., 2020; Wickramasinghe et al., 2021, 2022, 2024a, 2024b). Digital twins in healthcare have more broadly been viewed as mathematical models that are modelled as grey box, surrogate, and black box models (Wickramasinghe et al., 2021).

Grey Box Digital Twins

Grey box digital twins are typically based on well-studied principles, such as Physics (Wickramasinghe et al., 2021). For example, a Physics-based generic model of the human heart can be considered a grey model of the heart

(Hirschvogel et al., 2019). When such a model is calibrated to behave like the heart of a specific human, this becomes a grey box digital twin of the heart of that human.

Surrogate Digital Twins

Surrogate digital twins in healthcare are typically used for representative purposes (Wickramasinghe et al., 2021). They can represent the likes of devices, processes, or process flows in healthcare. As an example, consider the indicators of an electronic dashboard in an emergency department that show the real-time location of an ambulance with the state of its patient heading to trauma care (Croatti et al., 2020). That then becomes a surrogate digital twin of the ambulance and its patient. Such digital twins help the trauma care process flow by acting as a "representative model" that helps plan the right care. This can also help improve the efficiency and effectiveness of hospital or other healthcare workflows in general.

Black Box Digital Twins

Black box digital twins are those that are based on black box models discovered from data (Wickramasinghe et al., 2021). They are not governed by well-known principles, such as physics; rather, they are discovered from data (e.g., through machine learning or deep learning) to serve a purpose that is data intensive. Given the data intense and complex nature of the physical entities in healthcare such as patients, disease contexts, and healthcare workflows, it can be foreseen that black box digital twins will be the ones that find most powerful application in healthcare with an aim towards precision medicine and personalization of treatment (Wickramasinghe et al., 2021, 2022, 2023, 2024a, b). The integration of such black box models into existing clinical workflows as decision support tools have also been discussed (Wickramasinghe et al., 2023).

The Role of Neural Networks

Neural networks have become a cornerstone of modern artificial intelligence, particularly in deep learning applications which are often necessary for data-rich healthcare applications (Lu et al., 2017). The ability of neural networks to model complex, non-linear relationships makes neural networks ideal for black box modelling in healthcare applications through digital twins. In this section, various types of neural networks are explored by starting with the fundamental perceptron and delving into different types of neural networks and specific use cases in healthcare-related applications. The section is concluded with the latest advancements in liquid neural networks.

Perceptron

A perceptron is the simplest type of artificial neural network, consisting of a single layer of neurons. It was introduced by Frank Rosenblatt in 1957 and is designed for binary classification tasks. A perceptron takes multiple inputs, applies weights to them, sums them up, and passes the result through an activation function to produce a binary output.

Neural Network

A neural network is a collection of interconnected neurons organized in layers. It consists of an input layer, one or more hidden layers, and an output layer. Each neuron in a layer is connected to every neuron in the subsequent layer, forming a dense network typically performing weighted summation and activation functions. Neural networks are capable of learning from data through a process called training, where the weights and biases are adjusted to minimize the error between the predicted and actual outputs. Different types of neural networks can be formed and some of the common neural networks are discussed the subsections that follow along with some healthcare-related use cases available in literature.

Feedforward Neural Networks (FNNs)

Feedforward neural networks (FNNs) consist of an input layer, one or more hidden layers, and an output layer. Each neuron in a layer is connected to every neuron in the subsequent layer. The network learns by adjusting the weights of these connections based on the error of the predicted output compared to the expected training output. This process is known as training and typically involves backpropagation. In summary, in FNNs, information flows in one direction, from input to output, without cycles, and FNNs are simpler form of neural networks. Typical use cases for FNNs in healthcare can include predictive modelling for patient outcomes. For example, FNNs can be useful for predicting the likelihood of readmission for patients with chronic conditions by analysing historical health data.

The work by Sharma et al. (2024) discusses the transformative potential of Digital Twins (DTs) in healthcare, particularly for women's health issues like cervical cancer. The framework proposed in Sharma et al. (2024) focuses on automated cervical cancer detection using the SIPaKMeD dataset, which includes 1013 images from which 4103 cells have been extracted. The developed CervixNet classifier model detects and diagnoses cervical problems. Pre-trained recurrent neural networks (RNNs) have been used to extract 1172 features, and 792 features have been selected using principal component analysis (PCA). The model has achieved a high classification accuracy of 98.91%, especially with support vector machines (SVM). In this work, the proposed framework is interpreted as a DT, and it aligns with the interpretation by Wickramasinghe et al. (2021) as a black box DT of a healthcare workflow. This workflow helps in the detection and diagnosis of cervical cancer.

Based on such examples as the work of Sharma et al. (2024), several use cases of FNNs in healthcare digital twin applications can be foreseen. Some potential applications are summarized herein.

Predictive Analytics: FNNs can be used to predict patient outcomes based on historical health data. For instance, by analysing patient records, FNNs can predict the likelihood of disease recurrence, enabling proactive treatment plans.

Disease Diagnosis: In the context of disease detection such as cancer, FNNs can be trained on labelled datasets to classify inputs such as medical images as healthy or cancerous. This can significantly speed up the diagnostic process and improve accuracy.

Personalized Medicine: FNNs can be used to analyse a patient's information, such as genetic information, lifestyle, and medical history to recommend personalized treatment plans. This approach ensures that treatments are tailored to the individual, improving efficacy and reducing side-effects.

Medical Imaging: FNNs can be useful to enhance and interpret medical images, such as X-rays, MRIs, and CT scans. By learning from a large dataset of annotated images, FNNs can help identify patterns and anomalies that may be indicative of diseases.

Patient Monitoring: FNNs can process data from wearable devices to monitor vital signs in real time. This continuous monitoring can alert healthcare providers to any irregularities, allowing for timely intervention.

As such, FNNs can play a crucial role in healthcare applications through digital twin applications by enabling the likes of predictive analytics, disease diagnosis, personalized medicine, enhanced medical imaging, and patient monitoring. Their ability to learn from data and make accurate predictions makes them invaluable in creating a more efficient and effective healthcare system. As digital twin capabilities continue to evolve, the integration of FNNs can further enhance the capabilities of healthcare, leading to better patient outcomes and more personalized care.

Convolutional Neural Networks (CNNs)

Convolutional neural networks (CNNs) are a class of deep learning algorithms specifically designed for processing grid-like data, such as images. They consist of multiple layers, including convolutional layers, pooling layers, and fully connected layers. CNNs automatically and adaptively learn spatial hierarchies of features from input images, making them highly effective for image recognition and classification tasks.

CNNs work as follows. Convolutional layers apply convolution operations to the input, using filters to detect features such as edges, textures, and patterns. Pooling layers reduce the spatial dimensions of the data, retaining the most important features while reducing computational complexity. Fully connected layers connect every neuron in one layer to every neuron in the next layer, enabling the network to make final predictions based on the extracted features. CNNs can thus be used in healthcare-related Digital Twins for the purpose of analysing medical images.

The work by Ahmed et al. (2022) introduces a digital-twin-based smart healthcare system designed to enhance the efficiency and reliability of medical devices, particularly during the COVID-19 pandemic. This system integrates medical devices to collect real-time data on their health, configuration, and maintenance history. Additionally, it uses a deep-learning model based on a cascade recurrent convolution neural network (RCNN) architecture to analyse X-ray images for detecting COVID-19 infections. The RCNN model is trained in stages to improve accuracy and reduce false positives. The system has achieved a mean average precision rate of 0.94, demonstrating its effectiveness in detecting COVID-19.

CNNs can have various applications in healthcare applications as DTs. Some possible scenarios are summarized herein.

Analysing Medical Images: CNNs can be used to analyse X-ray, MRI, and CT scan images to detect various diseases such as cancer, or neurological disorders. By creating a digital twin of the imaging device, healthcare providers can monitor the device's performance and ensure accurate diagnostics as done by Ahmed et al. (2022).

Disease Detection and Diagnosis: CNNs can also analyse images like chest X-rays to detect signs of various infections. The digital twin of the diagnostic process can help in optimizing clinical workflows, increasing efficiency, and ensuring timely and accurate diagnosis.

Predictive Maintenance of Medical Devices: By integrating CNNs with digital twins of medical devices, healthcare providers can predict potential failures and schedule maintenance proactively. This reduces downtime and ensures that critical devices are optimally operational.

Personalized Treatment Plans: CNNs can be used to analyse patient-specific medical images to tailor treatment plans. For instance, in cancer, CNNs can help in identifying the exact location and the extent of tumours, allowing for precise radiation therapy planning.

Remote Monitoring and Telemedicine: CNNs can be used in telemedicine applications to analyse medical images sent by patients remotely. The digital twin of the telemedicine system can ensure that the images are processed accurately and that the system is functioning optimally.

CNNs as such can play a vital role in healthcare through digital twin applications by enhancing the likes of medical imaging analysis, disease detection, predictive maintenance, personalized treatment plans, and remote monitoring. Their ability to learn and extract meaningful features from complex medical images makes them useful in creating efficient and reliable decision support systems. The integration of CNNs in DTs thus can further revolutionize healthcare, leading to improved healthcare outcomes and efficient healthcare workflows and processes.

Recurrent Neural Networks (RNNs)

RNNs are a class of neural networks designed for processing sequential data. Unlike feedforward neural networks, RNNs have connections that form directed cycles, allowing them to maintain a memory of previous inputs. This makes them particularly suited for tasks where context and temporal dynamics are important.

RNNs process input sequences one element at a time, maintaining a hidden state that captures information about previous elements. This hidden state is updated at each time step based on the current input and the previous hidden state. Long Short-Term Memory (LSTM) networks are a type of RNN designed to overcome the limitations of traditional RNNs, such as the vanishing gradient problem. LSTMs use gates to control the flow of information, allowing them to capture long-term dependencies more effectively.

The work by Chakshu et al. (2021) attempts to address the challenge of improving healthcare infrastructure by leveraging the exponential rise in patient data. It proposes a method to create a cardiovascular digital twin using inverse analysis. Traditional methods for inverse analysis in linear problems are not effective for nonlinear systems like blood flow in the cardiovascular system. To overcome this, the authors propose a methodology using RNNs, specifically LSTM cells, to perform inverse analysis. By inputting blood pressure waveforms from three non-invasively accessible blood vessels (carotid, femoral, and brachial arteries), the system inversely calculates blood pressure waveforms in various vessels of the body. This approach is applied to detect abdominal aortic aneurysm (AAA) and assess its severity.

There can be various use cases of RNNs in healthcare as DTs and some possibilities are summarized herein.

Cardiovascular Monitoring and Analysis: As done by Chakshu et al. (2021), LSTM networks can be used to create cardiovascular DTs by analysing blood pressure waveforms. Such DTs can help in detecting conditions like AAA and assessing its severity. By continuously monitoring blood pressure data, such DTs can provide real-time insights into a patient's cardiovascular health.

Predictive Analytics for Chronic Diseases: RNNs can be used to predict the progression of chronic diseases such as diabetes or heart disease by analysing time-series data from patient records. A DT of the patient's health can simulate different scenarios and predict future health outcomes, enabling proactive interventions.

Personalized Treatment Plans: RNNs can be used to analyse a patient's historical health data to recommend personalized treatment plans. For instance, in managing hypertension, an RNN-based DT can be used to simulate the effects of different medications and lifestyle changes, helping doctors tailor treatments to an individual patient.

Remote Patient Monitoring: RNNs can be used to process data from wearable devices to monitor patients remotely. A DT of the patient's condition can be created to continuously analyse vital signs and detect anomalies, alerting healthcare providers about potential issues before they become critical.

Early Detection of Diseases: RNNs can be used to analyse patterns in patient data to detect diseases at an early stage. For example, an RNN-based DT can monitor changes in a patient's health metrics over time and identify early signs of conditions like Alzheimer's disease or Parkinson's disease.

RNNs can thus play a crucial role in healthcare applications through DTs, by enabling things like cardiovascular monitoring, predictive analytics, personalized treatment plans, remote patient monitoring, and early disease detection. The ability of RNNs to process sequential data and capture temporal dependencies makes them ideal for creating dynamic and responsive DTs. As healthcare continues to embrace digital transformation, the integration of RNNs can further enhance the capabilities of DTs, leading to improved healthcare outcomes and monitoring.

Autoencoders

Autoencoders are a type of neural network used for unsupervised learning. They consist of two main parts: an encoder that compresses the input data into a lower-dimensional representation and a decoder that reconstructs the original data from this compressed representation. The primary objective of an autoencoder is to learn an efficient encoding of the data, capturing the most important features while minimizing reconstruction error.

Encoders transforms the input data into a lower-dimensional latent space. Decoders reconstruct the input data from the latent representation. The Loss Function measures the difference between the original input and the reconstructed output, guiding the training process to minimize this error.

Autoencoders can have several use cases in healthcare as digital twin applications, and some are discussed herein.

Imputation of Missing Data: In healthcare, patient data often has missing values due to various reasons. Autoencoders can be used to impute these missing values by learning the relationships between different variables. For instance, an autoencoder can be used to replace missing variables with their reconstructed values, improving the accuracy of clinical forecasts.

Anomaly Detection: Autoencoders can be used to identify anomalies in patient data by learning the normal patterns and detecting deviations. In a DT representing a patient's conditions, autoencoders can flag unusual changes in clinical measurements or patient states, prompting further investigation and timely intervention.

Dimensionality Reduction: High-dimensional healthcare data can be challenging to analyse. Autoencoders can be used to reduce the dimensionality of data while preserving essential features. Such compressed representations can be used in DTs to simplify the analysis and visualization of complex patient datasets.

Feature Extraction: Autoencoders can be used to extract meaningful features from raw healthcare data, which can then be used for predictive modelling. In DTs, such features can help in accurately forecasting a patient's health trajectory and identifying potential risks.

Data Denoising: Health and medical data can be noisy due to measurement errors or external factors. Autoencoders can be trained to remove noise from data, providing cleaner and more reliable inputs for DTs. This enhances the quality of predictions and decision-making in DT healthcare applications.

Autoencoders can this play a crucial role in healthcare applications involving DTs by enabling the likes of data imputation, anomaly detection, dimensionality reduction, feature extraction, and data denoising. Their ability to learn efficient representations of complex data makes them useful in creating computationally efficient DTs.

Generative Adversarial Networks (GANs)

Generative Adversarial Networks (GANs) are a class of machine learning frameworks designed by Ian Goodfellow and his colleagues in 2014. GANs consist of two neural networks, the generator and the discriminator, which are trained simultaneously through adversarial processes. The generator creates synthetic data samples, while the discriminator evaluates them against real data samples, providing feedback to the generator to improve its outputs.

In GANs, the Generator produces synthetic data samples from random noise. The discriminator evaluates the authenticity of the generated samples compared to real data. In Adversarial Training, the generator and discriminator are trained in opposition, with the generator aiming to produce realistic samples and the discriminator striving to distinguish between real and fake samples.

There can be several use cases for GANs in healthcare as DTs, and some are summarized herein.

Medical Imaging Synthesis: GANs can be used to generate synthetic medical images, such as MRI or CT scans, to augment training datasets for diagnostic models. This is particularly useful in scenarios where obtaining large volumes of annotated medical images is challenging. By creating a DT of the imaging process, GANs can help improve the accuracy and robustness of diagnostic algorithms.

Data Augmentation: In clinical trials, GANs can be used to generate synthetic patient data that mimics real patient data. This can help in creating a DT of the patient population, enabling researchers to simulate various scenarios and improve the design and analysis of clinical trials.

Anomaly Detection: GANs can be trained to detect anomalies in medical data by learning the normal patterns and identifying deviations. For instance, a DT of a patient's condition can use GANs to flag unusual changes in vital signs or lab results, prompting further investigation.

Personalized Medicine: GANs can be used to generate personalized treatment plans by simulating how different treatments might affect a patient's condition. By creating a DT of a patient's profile, GANs can help doctors tailor treatments to the individual, improving outcomes and reducing side effects.

Drug Discovery: GANs can be used to generate the likes of new molecular structures for potential drug candidates. By creating a DT of the drug discovery process, GANs can accelerate the identification of promising compounds, reducing the time and cost associated with traditional drug development.

GANs can thus play a role in healthcare applications through DTs by enabling the likes of improvements in medical imaging synthesis, data augmentation, anomaly detection, personalized medicine, and drug discovery. Their ability processed by GANs to generate realistic synthetic data and model complex relationships makes them useful for creating DTs for various purposes in healthcare.

Liquid Neural Networks (LNNs)

Liquid neural networks (LNNs) are a recent advancement in neural network architecture. They are a type of recurrent neural networks that can adapt to changing conditions and learn from real-time data. Unlike traditional neural networks, liquid neural networks can adjust their parameters dynamically, making them highly suitable for applications requiring continuous learning and adaptation.

There are several possible use cases for LNNs including real-time patient monitoring. LNNs can continuously analyse data of patients, adapting to new information and providing timely alerts for critical conditions.

Among machine learning techniques, LNNs are highlighted for their unique ability to adapt dynamically to temporal data, offering robustness to noise and continuous learning capabilities. LNNs have been used to model DTs of patients having chronic diseases (Wickramasinghe & Ulapane, 2024).

LNNs have several attributes that can significantly enhance healthcare-related DT applications, and some are summarized herein.

Dynamic Adaptation: LNNs can adapt to temporal data, which is essential in healthcare where patient data is recorded over time. This allows for more accurate and timely predictions and interventions.

Robustness to Noise: Healthcare data often contains noise due to various factors like measurement errors or patient variability. The robustness shown by LNNs to noise ensures that the DTs remain reliable and accurate.

Continuous Learning: LNNs can learn continually from new data, making them ideal for managing chronic diseases where patient conditions can change over time. This continuous learning helps in updating DTs with the latest patient information, leading to better decision support.

Predictive Modelling: By using LNNs, DTs can predict disease progression and treatment outcomes, providing valuable insights for clinicians to make informed decisions.

Personalized Medicine: LNNs enable the creation of personalized DTs that reflect individual patient characteristics, leading to tailored treatment plans and improved patient outcomes.

In summary, LNNs offer a powerful tool for creating and managing digital twins in healthcare, providing dynamic, robust, and continuously learning models that can improve clinical decision-making and healthcare outcomes.

Conclusions

DTs are transforming industries by bridging the physical and digital worlds, enabling smarter, more efficient operations. As technology continues to advance, the applications and benefits of DTs will only expand, driving innovation and growth across various sectors, including healthcare. Neural networks play a pivotal role in black box modelling for healthcare applications through DTs. From the basic perceptron to advanced liquid neural networks, each type of neural network offers unique capabilities that can be leveraged to improve date driven decision-making in healthcare. This has the potential to entail in improved health outcomes in terms of improved patient outcomes, optimized and personalized treatment plans, and accelerated medical research, all while subscribing to value-based healthcare principles. As technology continues to evolve, the integration of neural networks in healthcare can thus lead to more innovative and effective solutions.

References

Ahmed, I., Ahmad, M., & Jeon, G. (2022). Integrating digital twins and deep learning for medical image analysis in the era of COVID-19. *Virtual Reality & Intelligent Hardware, 4*(4), 292–305.

Björnsson, B., Borrebaeck, C., Elander, N., Gasslander, T., Gawel, D. R., Gustafsson, M., Jörnsten, R., Lee, E. J., Li, X., & Lilja, S. (2020). Digital twins to personalize medicine. *Genome Medicine, 12*(1), 4.

Chakshu, N. K., Sazonov, I., & Nithiarasu, P. (2021). Towards enabling a cardiovascular digital twin for human systemic circulation using inverse analysis. *Biomechanics and Modeling in Mechanobiology, 20*(2), 449–465.

Croatti, A., Gabellini, M., Montagna, S., & Ricci, A. (2020). On the integration of agents and digital twins in healthcare. *Journal of Medical Systems, 44*(9), 161.

Hirschvogel, M., Jagschies, L., Maier, A., Wildhirt, S. M., & Gee, M. W. (2019). An in silico twin for epicardial augmentation of the failing heart. *International Journal for Numerical Methods in Biomedical Engineering, 35*(10), e3233.

Liu, Y., Zhang, L., Yang, Y., Zhou, L., Ren, L., Wang, F., Liu, R., Pang, Z., & Deen, M. J. (2019). A novel cloud-based framework for the elderly healthcare services using digital twin. *IEEE Access, 7*, 49088–49101.

Lu, L., Zheng, Y., Carneiro, G., & Yang, L. (2017). Deep learning and convolutional neural networks for medical image computing. *Advances in Computer Vision and Pattern Recognition, 10*, 978–973.

Marr, B. (2022). The Best Examples Of Digital Twins Everyone Should Know About; https://www.forbes.com/sites/bernardmarr/2022/06/20/the-best-examples-of-digital-twins-everyone-should-know-about/; date of last access: February 1, 2025.

Sharma, V., Kumar, A., & Sharma, K. (2024). Digital twin application in women's health: Cervical cancer diagnosis with CervixNet. *Cognitive Systems Research, 87*, 101264.

Siemens. (2025). Electrical Digital Twin; https://www.siemens.com/global/en/products/energy/grid-software/planning/electrical-digital-twin.html; date of last access: February 1, 2025.

Walker, A. (2023). Singapore's digital twin – from science fiction to hi-tech reality; https://infra.global/singapores-digital-twin-from-science-fiction-to-hi-tech-reality/; date of last access: February 1, 2025.

Wickramasinghe, N., Jayaraman, P. P., Forkan, A. R. M., Ulapane, N., Kaul, R., Vaughan, S., & Zelcer, J. (2021). A vision for leveraging the concept of digital twins to support the provision of personalized cancer care. *IEEE Internet Computing, 26*(5), 17–24.

Wickramasinghe, N., & Ulapane, N. (2024). Digital Twins of Patients: A Liquid Neural Network Interpretation. *ACIS 2024 Proceedings. 32.* https://aisel.aisnet.org/acis2024/32.

Wickramasinghe, N., Ulapane, N., Andargoli, A., Ossai, C., Shuakat, N., Nguyen, T., & Zelcer, J. (2022). Digital twins to enable better precision and personalized dementia care. *JAMIA Open, 5*(3), ooac072.

Wickramasinghe, N., Ulapane, N., Andargoli, A., Shuakat, N., Nguyen, T., Zelcer, J., & Vaughan, S. (2023). Digital twin of patient in clinical workflow. *Proceedings of the Royal Society of Victoria, 135*(2), 72–80.

Wickramasinghe, N., Ulapane, N., Sloane, E. B., & Gehlot, V. (2024a). Digital twins for more precise and personalized treatment. In *MEDINFO 2023—The future is accessible* (pp. 229–233). IOS Press.

Wickramasinghe, N., Ulapane, N., Zelcer, J., & Saffery, R. (2024b). Omics-based digital twins for personalised paediatric healthcare. *Studies in Health Technology and Informatics, 318*, 180–181.

Zorchenko, N., Tyupina, T., & Parshutin, M. (2024). Technologies used by general electric to create digital twins for energy industry. *Power Technology and Engineering, 58*(3), 521–526.

Part III

The How of Digital Twins

8

Digital Twins and Clinical Decision-Making

Introduction

As has been noted, digital twins are an engineering and manufacturing concept. When we look at applying this construct into the field of healthcare, a key area of interest is concerned with clinical decision-making. Clinical decision-making is an essential aspect in healthcare delivery, and it impacts both the quality of care provided and the cost or value of the care received. Thus, making prudent clinical decisions is of paramount importance, and digital solutions which facilitate this are of great merit.

In the beginning, digital twins were seen as virtual replicas of actual products, which served for knowledge forming, upkeep, and optimization of the real physical items. In manufacturing, digital twins became of significance when they were used as virtual representations of the complex systems to predict the future outcome of each process and also help in optimizing the production processes as well as facilitating predictive maintenance (Croatti et al., 2020). The initial achievement further inspired the expansion of the idea into various industries such as the aerospace, automotive, and energy.

Healthcare, with its imminent ecology of relationships and multiple factors of intimate interplay, represents an obvious area for the introduction of digital twins. Over the past few years, the digital twin concept has emerged as a critical parameter in providing the clinicians with the latest, and up to date information through data-driven insights and patient health and treatment outcomes (Alazab et al., 2022). This is made possible through cloning of a patient or a biological system, with continuously revised information obtained from multiple data sources. Such sources include the electronic health records (EHRs), medical images, genomic data, and others (Alazab et al., 2022).

Therefore, the power of digital twins in healthcare lies in reinventing the traditional healthcare models based on novel approaches that are not only focused on individuals but also predictive and proactive. The powerful features of digital twins, such as the use of advanced analytics, machine learning algorithms, and computational modelling, enable healthcare professionals to predict the development of diseases, plan the best method of treatment, and apply selected interventions to patients (Kaul et al., 2023).

As healthcare evolves into a digitalized industry, the adoption of digital microcosms is a transformative approach for medical decision-making. Instead of using only rearview data and generalized treatment methods,

DOI: 10.1201/9781003485971-11

physicians will now be able to use real-time, individual-specific information to give the kind of care that is more specific and better.

While the usage of digital twins in healthcare is not devoid of its difficulties, it brings certain opportunities that cannot be ignored. Still many ethical challenges need to be addressed, for example in the sphere of patients' confidentiality, data security, and consent to the use of this technology (Ahmadi-Assalemi et al., 2020). Moreover, technical impediments like interoperability, data aggregation, and algorithm biases hinder real-world implementation. All in all, the application of digital twin in healthcare is likely to make a significant difference. Digital twins will assist the clinicians to do more than just diagnosis, but also predict with precision and then recommend the right care with actionable insights. Thus, digital twins aid in improving the patient's life and saving life, i.e., both quality and quantity of life. However, in doing all this, it is good to understand that the road to the digital twins' development in the healthcare must be paved with a firm effort to guarantee high fidelity, ethical and trustworthy outputs which necessitates a responsible design.

Clinical Decision-Making

Decision-making can be categorized into three fundamental types: structured, semi-structured, and unstructured (Ulapane & Wickramasinghe, 2022). The fundamental aspect of structured decisions is that they contain clear procedures and well-defined problems, while semi-structured decisions involve a blend of structured frameworks or well-defined heuristics to form decisions and unstructured or complex elements. Finally, unstructured decisions are typically characterized by ambiguity and subjective interpretation and are focused on complex intractable problems. Hence, when it comes to support superior clinical decision-making, most assistance is required to be given to scenarios with semi-structured and unstructured decisions as these are the areas which tend to be most time consuming and more often than not lead to sub optimal decisions ensuing.

Background

Before it is possible to design and develop an appropriate integrated knowledge network that supports decision-making around an episode of care, it is necessary to first understand key, and often unique, aspects of the healthcare industry, the significant challenges, and the underlying healthcare value proposition. In sharp contrast to other industries, healthcare has a unique structure in which the receiver of the services (i.e., the patient) is often not the predominant payer for those services (i.e., the insurance company or government) (Wickramasinghe & Schaffer, 2010).

Further, healthcare interventions are typically complex and involve a variety of stakeholders including providers, payers, patients, and regulators (Wickramasinghe et al., 2008, 2009). This in turn leads to economic dilemmas such as moral hazard, orthogonal considerations pertaining to cost versus quality, and information asymmetry which in turn have the potential to create obstacles intentionally or not when trying to deliver efficient and effective healthcare (Boyd & Coram, 1976; von Lubitz & Wickramasinghe, 2006). To address these concerns and provide efficient, effective, and efficacious care delivery, relevant data, pertinent information, and germane knowledge play a vital role. However, these elements can only be obtained via the careful structure and design of a technology-enabled system which we have defined as the intelligence continuum (Alberts et al., 2001; Boyd, 1987; Cebrowski & Garstka, 1998).

To illustrate, we examine the arthroplasty episode of care starting with the evaluation of the operative procedure (Figure 8.1), the expansion of electronic medical records, interoperability, the possibility of data integration from previous episodic care environments, virtual care models, and increased patient engagement, has permitted an expansion of the datasets to include both facility and home care elements that will likely affect clinical processes (Schaffer et al., 2018). Integrating the patient's values, social determinants of health, health status and preferences into the model ensures optimization of addressing what matters most to the patient and what will be possible in the treatment paradigm of the episode of care.

Traditionally, the arthroplasty episode of care starts with awareness programmes that lead to access to care. Once the patient has an arthroplasty procedure the care is established with that surgeon and the patient often

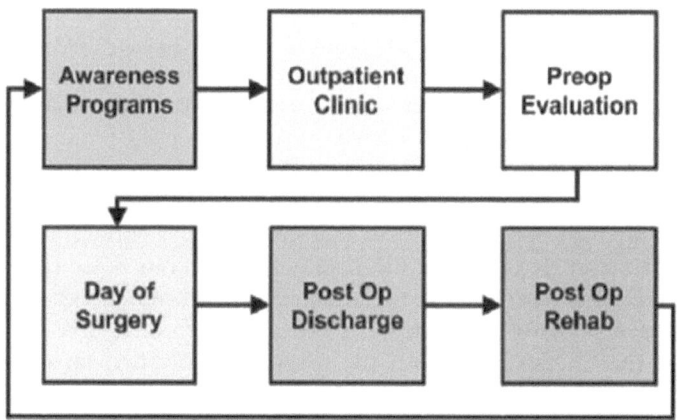

FIGURE 8.1
The episode of care in an arthroplasty context.

returns for a contralateral surgery or surgery on a different joint (adapted from Schaffer et al., 2018).

The intelligence continuum relies on multispectral inputs from patient data, established clinical practice guidelines, environmental data and psychosocial data, on which key analytics techniques, powered by the latest technologies and tools, are applied to identify critical patterns, insights, and factors to support expert judgement in deciding best practice to adopt along the clinical episode of care for the specific presenting patient (Wickramasinghe & Schaffer, 2010). In following such a precise and systematic protocol, it also becomes possible to simultaneously deliver on a healthcare value proposition of better access, quality, and value in the care delivery as well as ensure optimized clinical outcomes and patient satisfaction ensue. Integral to the successful application of the intelligence continuum is a process-centric perspective of knowledge creation which in turn leads to an integrated knowledge network (Wickramasinghe & Schaffer, 2010). This model leverages many aspects of a highly reliable organization. One such aspect is the reluctance to simplify. Taking into account a multitude of patient factors is complex. To be successful, knee arthroplasty decisions cannot be a "one-size-fits-all" process. Highly reliable processes embrace complex solutions for complex problems. Ongoing benchmarking and review of performance metrics will be needed to continuously improve and evolve the process (Hines et al., 2008).

The Process-Centric Perspective of Knowledge

A process-centric approach to knowledge creation serves to combine critical people-centric and technology-centric perspectives and at the same time emphasizes the dynamic and ongoing nature of the process (Wickramasinghe et al., 2009). This is particularly relevant for healthcare contexts as a healthcare intervention should not be viewed as a single moment in time but rather a progression of the patient along their care journey (Wickramasinghe et al., 2008). This process-centric perspective is grounded in the pioneering work of Boyd and his OODA (Observation followed by Orientation, then by Decision, and finally Action) loop, a conceptual framework that maps critical processes required to support rapid decision-making and extraction of essential and germane knowledge while filtering out extraneous noise (Alberts et al., 2000; Boyd, 1987; Cebrowski & Garstka, 1998; Wickramasinghe & Schaffer, 2006). As an instructor at the US Air Force Fighter Weapons School, Boyd developed the OODA loop with the premise that when an entity makes appropriate decisions the fastest, thereby completing the OODA loop in the shortest cycle time, they will become the victor (Alberts et al., 2000; Boyd, 1987; Cebrowski & Garstka, 1998). As in aviation, medical care involves continuous cycles of interaction between the patient and the treatment team to evaluate symptoms, diagnoses, treatments, and outcomes. Continuous improvement is necessary to ensure patient-centric evolution of the care process.

The OODA loop is based on a cycle of four interrelated stages essential to support critical analysis and rapid decision-making that revolve in both time and space: OODA (Alberts et al., 2000; Boyd, 1987; Cebrowski & Garstka, 1998). At the Observation and Orientation stages, implicit and explicit inputs are gathered or extracted from the environment (Observation) and then converted into coherent information (Orientation) (Alberts et al., 2000; Boyd, 1987; Cebrowski & Garstka, 1998). The latter determines the sequential determination (knowledge generation) and Action (practical implementation of knowledge) steps (Alberts et al., 2000; Boyd, 1987 Cebrowski & Garstka, 1998; Figure 8.2). The outcome of the Action stage then affects, in turn, the character of the starting point (Observation) of the next revolution in the forward progression of the continuous loop (Alberts et al., 2000; Boyd, 1987; Cebrowski & Garstka, 1998). Appropriate metrics are assessed and the cycle continues with a new cycle of observation (Wickramasinghe & Schaffer, 2006). In the patient context, a clinician completing the OODA loop in the shortest time will diagnose and treat the patient before situations change leading to an optimal clinical outcome (Wickramasinghe & Schaffer, 2010). As with fighter pilots, the OODA loop can be critical to patient survival.

This investigation establishes an integrated knowledge network framing to support optimal care management for knee arthroplasty care delivery. We contend it is only through such an approach that we can systematically deliver efficient, effective efficacious care that provides sound clinical

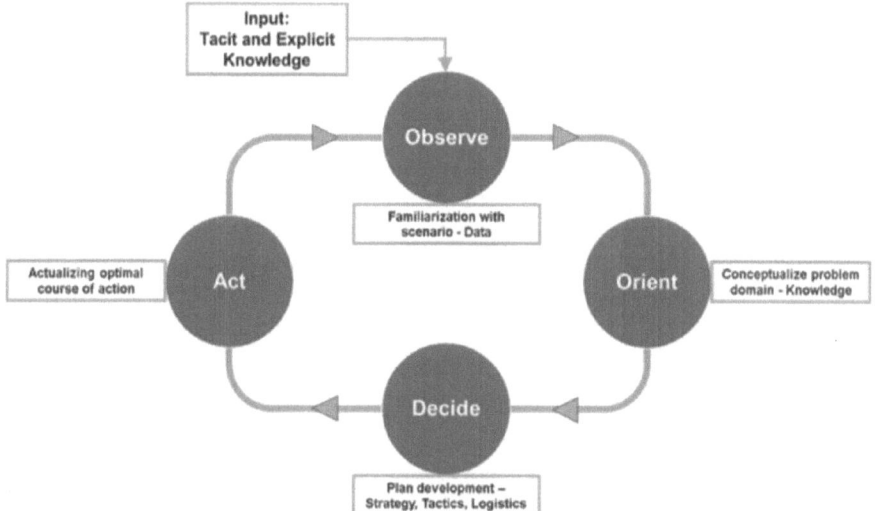

FIGURE 8.2
The OODA loop. Process Perspective of Knowledge Generation (adapted from Wickramasinghe & Schaffer, 2006).

outcomes and high patient satisfaction as well as supporting a healthcare value proposition of better access, quality, and value. It is against this background that we can then overlay the digital twin to provide superior, real-time decision-making and support. In this way, we not only serve to tighten or compress the decision-making time but also aided by the AI empowered digital twin provide more precise and personalized decisions.

Understanding Digital Twins

A digital twin is a virtual and dynamic model developed with fine detailed representative of a physical object or system that is directly connected and synchronized with its counterpart (Popa et al., 2021). To grasp digital twins, we have to analyse their base structures and synchronization ways as well as trace the transformative ability digital twins hold in the healthcare sector.

Components of Digital Twins

A digital twin comprises two fundamental components: the physical and the simulator. The physical model depicts the concrete, life-like representation of the actual entity or system that embodies its physical properties that give this its behaviours. This may include for instance a machine on a factory floor or the patient's physiological processes within a healthcare setting as examples. However, the virtual model provides a digital platform that is the virtual analog of the physical entity, incorporating information about its digital environment in the virtual environmental space. This digital twin enriched with data, algorithms, and simulations mimics the action of the real device and reveals its dynamics, properties, and responses (Bruynseels et al., 2018). By establishing advanced simulation and mathematical models, a virtual model could mimic the real-time system behaviour by simultaneously taking into account various components therein with considerable accuracy.

Synchronization Mechanisms

The main element of a digital twin is the smooth synchronized parallelism between physical and virtual model, maintaining precise synchronization of the digital twin with respect to the real-world model. The integration of the data is enhanced through various robust data collection mechanisms that constantly collect and update the data from different sources.

In the health sector, the patient's digital twin is aggregating data from many sources, such as EHRs, private devices (e.g., wearables), imaging scans, genetic information, and so on. By means of data integration pipelines and interoperability norms, these milieu of data are very often being integrated and consolidated and used in constructing a broad and multidimensional patient health status representation. For instance, digital twins can very easily monitor and collect irregular data with improved sensor technologies, IoT devices, and wireless communication networks. Through these technological developments, doctors and nurses are able to keep track of, analyse, and respond to constantly changing physiological parameters, so that they can promptly intervene and provide the personalized treatment that is needed.

Application of Digital Twins in Healthcare

In healthcare, the digital twin application is multi-faceted and ranges from the healthcare processes to the scientific research. It presents a new way of optimizing and rethinking the clinical decision-making, patients care, and medical research processes (Angulo et al., 2020). An important application of this approach is the prediction of disease progression, estimating treatment results, and identification personalized risk factors which can be performed by digital twins giving a chance to clinicians to do so in advance.

By way of example, take a person who has received a chronic illness diagnosis like diabetes for instance. Physicians can experiment with the patient's avatar so that they can create several scenarios of treatment, determine future impact of various interventions, and personally adjust the plan for optimal effects with minimum risk. On the other hand, digital twins also allow the patients to actively join the process by favouring personalized recognition, applicable suggestions, and self-management tools.

In addition, digital twins take on a vital role in medical education, training, as well as simulation once again. Healthcare professionals can realize digital twins as a great tool to run complicated healthcare procedures, practise the skills of performing surgeries, and improve their clinical proficiency without any worries in the virtual environment (Rivera et al., 2019). Besides that, digital twins are really useful for medical researchers to conduct virtual clinical trials, digitalize disease mechanisms, and will accelerate the discovery of new treatments and interventions.

Basically, digital twins in healthcare will contribute to a significant breakthrough in the journey to personalized medicine and precision medicine delivery. With real-time patient data synched together with computational modelling and statistical analysis, digital twins bring in a revolutionary paradigm in medical decision-making that crosses several medical areas.

The Predicting Model of Outcomes for Patients

In the medical sector, the predictive modelling for patient results is one of the crucial use of the digital twins. Leveraging past patient information, physiological changes, as well as the path of progression in diseases, digital twins produce highly accurate prediction of the status of individual patients. For an instance, the situation of the long-term illnesses like the cardiovascular and diabetes disorders, digital twins can examine the timeline and future complications such as the heart attacks or strokes. Through the usage of predictive analytics, clinicians get the chance to act in a timely manner with ensuring timely implementation of actions aimed at alleviating risks and achieves better outcomes.

On the other hand, digital twins can facilitate healthcare providers to identify best conditions that signal erroneous events or aggravation of diseases. Through constant tracking of key biomarkers, physiological variables, and behavioural trends, digital twins expand the early warning system, giving clinicians a signal on any deviation from norms and thus preceding action (Elkefi & Asan, 2022). For instance, heart patients with digital twins can monitor any signals of harm and so the system can appropriately adjust the medication regimens or recommend lifestyle modifications as necessary to prevent hospitalization.

Personalized Treatment Plans

Another more developing application of digital twins in health is the development of personalized treatment regimens designed for each patient's uniqueness in physiological properties, genetic characteristics, and clinical history. Usually, the traditional approach to medical treatment uses uniform therapy protocols which have in consideration the fact that not all patients will respond to the treatment equally, and the disease process of the different patients may be different. Digital twins could be the means to do this because clinicians can now customize strategies according to current data and simulations that are present (Venkatesh et al., 2024).

In the oncology field, digital twins can blend genomic data and phenotypic characteristics with data on the treatment response, and as a result, it can guide the choice of targeted therapies or immunotherapies. Digital twins dig down the effectiveness of various treatment alternatives in silo and give authority to the oncologist to tune up the therapy route, reduce the toxicity side effects, and enhance the therapeutic efficacy specifically for each patient. For instance, in pharmacogenomics, digital twins can predict individual drug responses based on genetic polymorphisms which may ultimately help to prescribe the most effective medicine with the least amount of risk (De Maeyer & Markopoulos, 2021).

Simulation of Medical Procedures

Digital twins are not only helpful from the point of view of predictive modelling and individualized treatment planning, but they also provide a lot of useful information associated with the procedure of virtual simulations of medical interventions. From the surgical simulator to the virtual trial, as digital twins are applied, clinicians and researchers gain experience by probing the possible outcomes of medical interventions in a safe digital environment. Digital twins are able to duplicate the bodily variations of patient anatomy and pathology, so this makes the preoperative planning, procedural iteration, and device optimization more efficient. This will improve patient safety and procedural outcomes.

For instance, in neurosurgery, digital twins can model the brain functioning as well as the benefits and negative outcomes of the procedures. This gives the neurosurgeon a better chance at visualizing critical anatomy, planning out the most ideal trajectories and being able to foresee the challenges. Using patient specific in vivo data with computer models of brain anatomy and biomechanics, surgeons can be guided through complex surgical procedures with accuracy and conviction, which are the critical elements for getting successful results. Also, in the field of medical device development, digital twins act as the global virtual testing grounds for assessment of device performance, tuning of design parameters, and validation of safety and effectiveness before clinical trials.

Integration of Digital Twins into Clinical Decision-Making

Not only will the incorporation of digital twins into evidence-based medicine accelerate the pace of change in healthcare, but it will also have a tremendously significant impact on the quality of care patients receive. For the accomplishment of the integration of AI into the healthcare system smoothly, some crucial elements should be considered such as painless data gathering, the use of AI algorithms, and the thoughtful ethic concerns of patient data confidentiality and privacy (Huang et al., 2022).

The Automatic Data Collection and Integration of All the Stages

The key building blocks of digital twin technology are the acquisition and linkage of data from a variety of sources, such as EHR, wearable devices, medical imaging, and other health monitoring systems. These sources constitute of vital pieces of information that will enable the health workers to be sure of a patient's health status. The combination of all these sources gives a complete health picture of a patient.

EHR, in turn, are the places where clinical data of patients can be stored systematically and this information includes demographic data, medical history, diagnoses, medications, and treatment plans. The combination of EHR information with the digital models called digital twins allows the clinicians easy access and real-time use of the comprehensive information about the patient, which in turn gives them an opportunity to make better-informed decisions on the spot.

When it comes to devices such as heart rate monitors, blood pressure monitors, and movement trackers, combining the data they provide with digital twin can help physicians calculate longitudinal graphs and real-time alerts and therefore have an early detection of anomalies and timely interventions. Imaging techniques that can display this type of information might include X-rays, MRIs, and CT scans. This makes the doctor able to see delicate internal structures such as the brain, heart, and kidneys in greater detail. Bringing in imaging data into digital twins allows the clinicians to use the visuals in tracking the progression of the disease, assess the efficiency of the treatment, and help them plan the surgical intervention with more precision.

Utilization of AI and Machine Learning Algorithms

The massive amount of data produced by digital twins certainly becomes a daunting task in the execution, analysis, and interpretation. By automating the process of data analysis, identifying patterns and providing actionable insights, AI and machine learning algorithms play a key role in assisting clinicians to answer this challenge. With the help of machine learning algorithms, pattern recognition in complex data can be performed to find possible links, predict patient outcomes, and choose the best treatment for the patient. With the use of historical patients' data, and machine learning models, it becomes possible to recognize risk factors, predict disease course and recommend customized interventions adapted to individual's character-istics for each patient.

Natural language processing (NLP) algorithms extract from unstructured clinical notes and narrative reports contained within the EHR the nuanced insights necessary to make objective and evidence-based decisions. Via the process of text analysis, NLP algorithms can detect clinical concepts, extract pertinent data, and accordingly use it for the purpose of integration of the textual data into digital twins for a differential and exhaustive examination.

Basically, AI-driven algorithm systems serve as real-time decision support systems to furnish practitioners with the actionable insights and preferences required at the time of medical care. For this, systems can look at real-time patient data and clinical guidelines, to get triggers to potential adverse events, recommend evidence-based interventions, and help clinicians in their decision-making.

Challenges and Considerations

While the possible benefits of digital twins in healthcare are huge, the broad implementation or their application comes with various challenges and con-ditions that should be taken into account. However, the major issues are those associated with data security and privacy. One more is that of interoperabil-ity. The unification of different types of data sources, for example, the elec-tronic health registries, the wearable sensors, and the genomic record banks, gives rise to privacy issues, such as patient confidentiality, data breaches, and compliance of the research data with the regulations. Furthermore, in order to reap the full benefits of digital twin platforms in clinical proceedings, the provision of smooth interoperability of digital twin platforms with other healthcare information technology systems is of immeasurable importance.

Furthermore, there is the challenge of developing reliable and validated digital twin models as well as achieving effective collaborations within inter-disciplinary domains of clinicians, data scientists, engineers, and regulatory experts. Conducting precision validation studies and test protocols that are sturdy as well as conducting reporting standards that are transparent is also a challenge to some extent.

The scalability, reliability, and performance of digital twins can also demand robust infrastructural investment which can be costly to acquire and maintain. Developing digital twin designs with robust computational set-up, parallel computing technologies, and data analytics capabilities for the processing of massive data chunks of healthcare data is a must for effi-cient prediction. However, having this realized will require a lot of cash which can be a challenge to many organizations.

Ethical Considerations: Patient Data Security and Confidentiality Issues

More and more healthcare entities today start to make use of digital twins for clinical decision-making, which calls for security and privacy of patient data. Such ethical issues associated with patient data security and privacy need to be rigorously acknowledged to preserve the trust of the patient and to comply with the regulatory framework. Data encryption and access controls serve as a means of making sure that patient data doesn't get into unauthorized users' hands and that it remains confidential throughout its life cycle. Through the process of adopting reliable encryption algorithms and permission levels, health organizations could reduce the risk of data leakage and illegal disclosure while making use of digital twins (Huang et al., 2022).

Anonymity and de-identification principles can be used to remove from risk of identification any patient data without diminishing the value of the data for research and analysis purposes. For instance, healthcare organizations could de-identify sensitive data items including patient names, social security numbers and dates of birth through anonymization. It would help decrease the risk of re-identification and also protect patient anonymity.

Transparency and informed consent are two fundamental tenets that are imperative for the ethical utilization of patients' data for digital twins. It is the responsibility of healthcare providers to outline the purpose of data collection and analysis in a manner that is understandable and free of ambiguity to patients (Meijer et al., 2023). Obtaining an informed consent from the patients helps them to realize that they have consented to the researchers to utilize their data for the purpose of clinical decision-making.

Routine auditing and compliance monitoring serve as the centre pin of the process to make sure that the required ethics standards and regulations are always followed. This can be apparent through periodical audit of data on files, checking of compliance with data security policies together with taking corrective actions, if necessary, in healthcare.

Future Directions and Challenges

Digital twin advancements in healthcare biotechnology are set to cover a wide range of opportunities, but, unfortunately, at the same time, they may lead to some serious hurdles that will have to be studied very carefully. In the coming years, this technology will continue to do its magic in various areas which include advancement and problems to be tackled to unleash its full power.

Better Interoperability among Healthcare Systems

There is no doubt that the interoperability of information technology among different medical systems will be the number one goal for the medical digital twin in the future. The health data we have today tends to be scattered in unconnected storage systems hindering interoperability between entities like healthcare providers, laboratories, clinics, and pharmacies. The open development and implementation of standardized data formats, protocols, and application systems interfaces (APIs) is necessary to ensure the digital twins interoperability and the smooth integration of digital twins in the current healthcare ecosystems.

In addition, interoperability goes beyond technical considerations but extends its impact to include law, regulation, and organization. Creating a common regulatory framework and offering more incentives for stakeholders from various segments of the healthcare sector are the crucial measures to be carried out before the population as a whole starts using digital twins actively.

Improved AI Algorithms Are an Advantage of Big Data Analysis

For artificial intelligence in healthcare to be fully realized, its researchers must continue to debug existing algorithms, devise new methodologies, and control the biases that AI engenders in its decision-making systems. On top of this, it is crucial to carry out the process that guarantees AI algorithms transparency, interpretability, and ethical integrity due to their crucial importance in healthcare. Current advances which include liquid neural networks hold the promise of faster and adaptive systems that do not require as large storage and are more agile. What is clear is that as technology and AI advances so too will the level of sophistication and predictive power of the developed digital twins.

Workforce Training and Capacity Development

Along with growing integration of digital twins into clinical practice, the need to train and upskill workers, as well as to enhance their capacity, arises as one of the key areas of focus to make sure that the use of digital twin technologies in healthcare settings is effective and sustainable. Medical professionals should be ready to receive the necessary knowledge, skills, and competencies to digital twins' application for clinical processes, clinical workflows, and the decision-making processes.

That collaboration between different disciplines is also necessary to realize the full benefit of digital twins. medical care Clinicians, data scientists, informaticians, engineers, and all the healthcare stakeholders need to cooperate closely so as to co-create, define, implement and test digital twin solutions that are better suited to solve clinical issues, improve patient care and motivate the level of innovation in healthcare delivery.

Also, one should strive to engage in continuous professional development, lifelong learning, and skills training in order to run in tandem with the fast-paced technological advancements and applied uses of digital twin technologies in healthcare. Training courses, workshops, and educational resources designed for healthcare professionals based on their specific needs can give them the required skills to use digital twins seamlessly and incorporate advanced analytics into their medications which will in turn, enhance their practice.

To sum up, there is a great potential for digital twins in healthcare to improve patient care, motivate innovation, and even to change healthcare delivery working mechanisms. While we acknowledge that biotechnology can contribute to the solution, it is, however, only part of the whole process. It remains to be seen whether bioethics can produce positive results or not. Combining efforts interdisciplinarity, partnerships, and persistent innovation in healthcare organizations makes it possible to embrace the full potential of digital twins to enhance patient outcomes, rigorous decision-making processes and to even reshape healthcare delivery.

Value-Based Healthcare and Enhanced Recovery after Surgery

As the challenges of providing quality care and access to care for all at an appropriate value increases most especially as we come out of COVID-19, two key paradigms are becoming more and more significant; namely, (1) the provision of value-based care and (2) ensuring enhanced recovery after surgery (ERAS). Both are related in so far as they are both fulfilled when sound clinical decision-making occurs. When prudent prevention, triage and perioperative steps are taken and a successful surgery occurs the probability of enhanced recovery after the surgery is significantly higher. This also translates into a higher value outcome. As we have discussed in the preceding section, superior clinical decision-making can be greatly enabled through the incorporation of digital twins. Thus, we contend that one of the most prudent ways to support the two key paradigms today, i.e., value case care and ERAS, is to incorporate digital twins into all clinical decision-making and most especially complex clinical decision-making.

Conclusion

The digital twin is at the very front of technological development and is perhaps one of the best breakthroughs in the field of health that can change the clinical decision-making in healthcare. Digital twins empower user with the combined skills of collecting real-time data and smart AI algorithms to revolutionize the medical field by improving the treatment processes and launching new medical scientific research. While digital twins enjoy the great benefits of yielding a comprehensive, data-informed picture of patient conditions as well as the treatment options available, clinicians stand to benefit by having this knowledge at their disposal. Digital twins are refreshed on an ongoing basis by creating digital representations of physical entities. This makes them into an interactive platform where huge amounts of diverse data can be processed. This allows the clinicians to make personalized decisions with the exact needs of each patient in mind, and therefore, highly effective treatments are achieved and favourable results are obtained.

However, digital twins are not only confined to patients' well-being. They could also be used to bring about notable progress in medical research and innovation. Through reflecting the variety of conditions and determining the expected results, digital twins are able to discover new treatment approaches, adjust existing methods, and hurry up the evolution of new medicines. Thus, the efficiency of individual patients by providing personalized care is not only enhanced but also the digital twins promote the development of the scientific society in terms of expanding the understanding of the disease mechanisms and the treatment responses.

For the digital twin technology in healthcare to be implemented on the large scale, comprehensive research and development, as well as joint efforts in innovation and cooperation, are indispensable. A constant investment in upgrading technological functionality and networking, together with the incorporation of digital twins into the clinical practice, has to be done to bolster the capabilities of these models. However, collaborative approach between the healthcare providers, researchers, tech professionals, and policy-makers is extremely vital to combat the complicated matters related to data integration, privacy, and compliance of regulations. It is clear that digital twins are at their infancy and as they develop in sophistication and computational power they will become more and more essential in the support of superior, personalized yet precise clinical decision-making.

References

Ahmadi-Assalemi, G., Al-Khateeb, H., Maple, C., Epiphaniou, G., Alhaboby, Z. A., Alkaabi, S., & Alhaboby, D. (2020). Digital twins for precision healthcare. In H. Jahankhani, S. Kendzierskyj, N. Chelvachandran, & J. Ibarra (Eds.), *Cyber defence in the age of AI, Smart societies and augmented humanity* (pp. 133–158). Springer.

Alazab, M., Khan, L. U., Koppu, S., Ramu, S. P., Iyapparaja, M., Boobalan, P., Baker, T., Maddikunta, P. K. R., Gadekallu, T. R., & Aljuhani, A. (2022). Digital twins for healthcare 4.0—Recent advances, architecture, and open challenges. *IEEE Consumer Electronics Magazine, 12*(6), 29–37.

Alberts, D. S., Garstka, J. J., Hayes, R. E., & Signori, D. A. (2001). *Understanding information age warfare.* CCRP. http://www.dodccrp.org/files/Alberts_UIAW.pdf

Angulo, C., Gonzalez-Abril, L., Raya, C., & Ortega, J. A. (2020, April). A proposal to evolving towards digital twins in healthcare. In *International work-conference on bioinformatics and biomedical engineering* (pp. 418–426). Springer International Publishing.

Boyd, J. R., in Patterns of Conflict (1987) Unpublished briefing, accessible as "Essence of Winning and Losing," http://www.d-n-i.net.

Boyd, J. R., & Coram, R. (1976). *Destruction and creation.* "Boyd," Little, Brown & Co.

Bruynseels, K., Santoni de Sio, F., & Van den Hoven, J. (2018). Digital twins in health care: Ethical implications of an emerging engineering paradigm. *Frontiers in Genetics, 9,* 320848.

Cebrowski, A. K., & Garstka, J. J. (1998). Network-centric warfare: Its origin and future. *US Naval Institute Proceedings, 1,* 28–35.

Croatti, A., Gabellini, M., Montagna, S., & Ricci, A. (2020). On the integration of agents and digital twins in healthcare. *Journal of Medical Systems, 44*(9), 161.

De Maeyer, C., & Markopoulos, P. (2021, July). Future outlook on the materialisation, expectations and implementation of Digital Twins in healthcare. In *34th British HCI conference* (pp. 180–191). BCS Learning & Development.

Elkefi, S., & Asan, O. (2022). Digital twins for managing health care systems: Rapid literature review. *Journal of Medical Internet Research, 24*(8), e37641.

Steve Hines, Katie Luna, Jennifer Lofthus, Michael Marquardt, and Dana Stelmokas. (2008, April). Becoming a high reliability organization: Operational advice for hospital leaders. AHRQ Publication No. 08-0022. Agency for Healthcare Research and Quality.

Huang, P. H., Kim, K. H., & Schermer, M. (2022). Ethical issues of digital twins for personalized health care service: Preliminary mapping study. *Journal of Medical Internet Research, 24*(1), e33081.

Kaul, R., Ossai, C., Forkan, A. R. M., Jayaraman, P. P., Zelcer, J., Vaughan, S., & Wickramasinghe, N. (2023). The role of AI for developing digital twins in healthcare: The case of cancer care. *Wiley Interdisciplinary Reviews: Data Mining and Knowledge Discovery, 13*(1), e1480.

Meijer, C., Uh, H. W., & El Bouhaddani, S. (2023). Digital twins in healthcare: Methodological challenges and opportunities. *Journal of Personalized Medicine, 13*(10), 1522.

Popa, E. O., van Hilten, M., Oosterkamp, E., & Bogaardt, M. J. (2021). The use of digital twins in healthcare: Socio-ethical benefits and socio-ethical risks. *Life Sciences, Society and Policy, 17*(1), 25.

Rivera, L. F., Jiménez, M., Angara, P., Villegas, N. M., Tamura, G., & Müller, H. A. (2019, November). Towards continuous monitoring in personalized healthcare through digital twins. In *Proceedings of the 29th annual international conference on computer science and software engineering* (pp. 329–335). IBM Corp.

Schaffer, J. L., Rasmussen, P. A., & Faiman, M. R. (2018). The emergence of distance health technologies. *Journal of Arthroplasty, 33,* 2345–2351.

Ulapane, N., & Wickramasinghe, N. (2022). Scoping Mobile clinical decision support systems to enhance design and recording of usage data effectively: A suggested approach. In *Digital disruption in healthcare* (pp. 209–225). Springer.

Venkatesh, K. P., Brito, G., & Kamel Boulos, M. N. (2024). Health digital twins in life science and health care innovation. *Annual Review of Pharmacology and Toxicology, 64,* 159–170.

von Lubitz, D., & Wickramasinghe, N. (2006). Healthcare and technology: The doctrine of network-centric healthcare. *International Journal of Electronic Healthcare, 4,* 322–344.

Wickramasinghe, N., Bali, R., Lehany, B., Gibbons, C., & Schaffer, J. L. (2009). *Health care knowledge management primer.* Routledge.

Wickramasinghe, N., & Schaffer, J. L. (2006). Creating knowledge driven healthcare processes with the intelligence continuum. *International Journal of Electronic Healthcare, 2,* 164–174.

Wickramasinghe, N., & Schaffer, J. (2010). Realizing Value Driven Patient Centric Healthcare Delivery Through Technology, IBM Center for the Business of Government, http://www.businessofgovernment.org/report/realizing-value-driven-e-health-solutions (accessed February 2020).

Wickramasinghe, N., Schaffer, J. L., & Bali, R. (2008). The health care intelligence continuum: Key model for enabling KM initiatives and realising the full potential of SMT in healthcare delivery. *International Journal of Biomedical Engineering and Technology, 1,* 415–427.

9

Application of Digital Twins in Healthcare Processes

Introduction

Digital twin is a game-changing technology that has progressed from its original industrial use to become a novel concept in the area of healthcare optimization. By definition, digital twin can be described as a virtual duplicate of a physical object, possesses the same real attributes, manifests the same behaviours, and works together with physical entities or systems to accomplish particular objectives. This technology works as a tool in healthcare to reflect numerous components such as individuals, medical devices, and whole healthcare facilities using data-based decision-making.

The role of digital twins in healthcare is without a doubt nothing to be overlooked. Healthcare systems are intrinsically complicated, with their unique features that include the complex processes, many actors, and the critical moments of decisions. The advent of the ability to construct digital copies of these systems would undoubtedly offer immense benefits. Through this technology, healthcare professionals will have the opportunity to explore the patients' health status, reorganize workflow processes, and promote optimal resource utilization. The technology can also make real-time monitoring and analysis possible. This helps in the prevention of crises and personalized care delivery. However, for this to be possible, digital twin technology has to combine multiple features, such as the use of robust IT infrastructure and various datasets. This leads to harmonization of scattered datasets which ultimately define individualized or personalized approaches in the healthcare delivery.

As healthcare systems grapple with challenges such as rising costs, population aging, and evolving disease patterns, the need for innovative solutions has never been more urgent. Digital twins offer a paradigm shift in how healthcare processes are conceptualized, managed, and optimized. By leveraging digital twins, healthcare organizations can unlock new efficiencies, improve patient outcomes, and ultimately, transform the healthcare landscape. To better understand healthcare processes and techniques to make these processes more lean and efficient it is necessary to understand lean thinking, total quality management (TQM), and other related concepts.

DOI: 10.1201/9781003485971-12

Lean Thinking

Lean thinking, which developed from lean manufacturing or the Toyota Production System (TPS), is centred around elimination of waste and preserving value. Lean became especially important, some may go so far to say a fad, in manufacturing in the 1990s. So why in the 21st century might the principles of lean be relevant to healthcare? In order to understand this, we need to recognize that healthcare delivery today is facing many pressures much like much of the manufacturing industries in the 1990s. Specifically, healthcare delivery today throughout the world is in a conundrum. Escalating costs, aging populations, increase in chronic diseases and growth in medical technology solutions are some of the major challenges with which all healthcare systems must contend. Governments, policymakers, and clinicians are all in agreement that healthcare reform is necessary and new strategies, protocols, and procedures are required if healthcare delivery is to in fact provide appropriate access, quality, and value to patients and the community at large. Most are turning to digital solutions empowered by artificial intelligence (AI) as the silver bullet. However, this is only part of the solution. The other part of the solution lies in the embracement of leading management principles and techniques which support and enable lean thinking and value creation and generation. The following serves to introduce the key concepts in lean thinking as relevant for healthcare.

TQM and Kaizen

Integral to lean manufacturing are the concepts of TQM and Kaizen. Both concepts focus on continuous improvements, the importance of process and performance to achieve positive outcomes and the key role of people. TQM is a philosophy (Deming, 1986) while Kaizen is a technique. The later tends to focus on quality and customer satisfaction while the latter takes a top-down approach and focuses on small incremental stages.

TQM

While there are many definitions of TQM simply stated TQM is a continuous quality improvement approach (Nawar, 2008). It has also been described as a total organization approach (Oakland, 2012), an effort to improve the whole organization's competitiveness, effectiveness, and structure (Dale, 1999) and requires the mutual co-operation of management, employees, suppliers, and customers (Dale, 1999). Many scholars and proponents (Deming, 1986; Juran, 1993; Scholtes, 1992) have noted that TQM and more especially a quality focus are important for long-term success.

Kaizen

In contrast to TQM Kaizen is a technique (Imai, 1997). Kaizen means continuous improvement and assumes managers and employees work together to achieve this and such efforts do not require tremendous resources.

The key elements of Kaisen include:

1. Team work
2. Personal discipline
3. Improved morale
4. Quality circles
5. Suggestions for improvement
6. Elimination of wastes and inefficiency
7. The 5S framework (Saleem et al., 2012) – (1) Seiri (sorting out), (2) Seiton (systematic arrangement), (3) Seiso (spic and span), Seiketsu (standardizing) and Shitsuke (self-discipline).

In addition to the elements of Kaizen, Kaizen techniques can be applied at three different levels:

1. Individual versus team
2. Day-to-day versus special events
3. Process level versus sub-process level

In addition to the philosophy of lean and the techniques of Kaizen other complementary management methodologies and theories include six sigma and constraints management. The following briefly looks at each in turn.

Six Sigma

Six sigma has emerged as a primary vehicle for improving both manufacturing and service processes (Inozu et al., 2012). Specifically, "six sigma is a rigorous and systematic methodology that utilizes information (management by facts) and statistical analysis to measure and improve a company's operational performance, practices and systems by identifying and preventing 'defects' in manufacturing and service–related processes in order to anticipate and exceed expectations of all stakeholders to accomplish effectiveness" (Inozu et al., 2012, p. 20). A five-step define-measure-analyse-improve-control (DMAIC) methodology is used where each step outlines distinct and key activities that must be performed as follows:

1. Define the business issue
2. Measure the process

3. Analyse the data and verify root causes of variation

4. Improve the process

5. Control the process and sustain improvements

Six sigma has the power to save healthcare millions of dollars. Usually this is achieved by combining the key components of six sigma with one of the major principles of Lean; namely the seven deadly wastes.

Constraints Management

The last complementary methodology that will be presented in this chapter is that of constraints management. Constraints management is made up of a suite of techniques used in operations and supply chain management. The key being to enable a systematic approach to manage complex organizations by identifying and controlling key leverage points within the system. Some of the basic constraint types include:

1. Market

2. Resources

3. Materials

4. Supplier/vendor

5. Financial

6. Knowledge/competence

7. Policy

As noted, healthcare delivery today is under pressure to deliver high-quality outcomes, contain costs as well as contend with other challenges such as increase in chronic diseases and the impact of technology advances on healthcare delivery. All are agreed that healthcare reform is necessary, and we are witnessing in all Organization for Economic Cooperation and Development (OECD) countries a focus on healthcare reform with a key enabler being a myriad of digital health solutions. The preceding has introduced the principles of lean thinking and other complementary concepts all aimed at effecting more efficient and effective operations to ensue. These tools and techniques have proved their value in the manu-facturing sector and can provide equally beneficial results if applied to the healthcare sector. It is therefore essential that practitioners and research-ers alike try to embrace lean principles and related concepts as they set about designing and developing new healthcare initiatives. However, it is the thesis of this chapter that we can leverage the benefits even further by combining digital twins with the adoption of lean principles and the other aforementioned concepts.

Components of Digital Twins

At its core, digital twin comprises three fundamental components: the physical module, the virtual counterpart, and the data fusion layer.

The Physical Entity

A physical entity symbolizes the material representation of the simulation. Within the field of medicine this whole notion could include quite a large part like patients, medical equipment, medicines, and entire healthcare facilities. The particular attributes of each element, including the behaviour and interactions, determine its position and function within a healthcare system's full network. As an example, the patient's physical entity would involve data such as age, medical history, and the medications that they are taking as well as their ongoing treatment. Through the able representation of these physicality, digital twins pave a way for realistic simulation and data-driven decision-making procedure regarding healthcare processes.

The Virtual Model

The virtual model can be considered just the digital version of the physical one, in which all significant characteristics, behaviour, and dynamics that are associated with it are embedded. In healthcare, virtual representatives can assume different forms, depending on the kind of entity they embody. The patient simulators can be made to have physiological simulations, disease models, and treatment algorithms as they look to mimic the intricacies of the human body and disease. These digital models let healthcare providers be in track on patient health, forecast disease progression, and find out admission strategy extemporaneously. Similarly, device digital twins may include behaviour models, failure modes, and performance metrics to simulate the operation and maintenance of medical equipment. By leveraging virtual models, healthcare organizations can identify potential issues, optimize workflows, and ensure the reliable operation of critical medical devices.

The Data Integration Layer

The data integration layer acts as a middle area in the process of connecting the physical entity with the digital model and, therefore, enables transfer of knowledge and information in real time. This layer of a healthcare network has its data sources spread across diverse areas including sensors, electronic health records (EHRs), medical imagery, and laboratory tests. The data integration layer provides a comprehensive view of the complexities involved in the model by incorporating, analysing, and interpreting data from these sources into the virtual model in a timely and pertinent manner. In this regard, sensors inside wearables can record vital signs of the patient, body movements, and environmental condition which are later on included in the digital twin to ensure further monitoring and analysis. And just like EHR systems do, the virtual models use patient records, treatment histories, and diagnostic information that boost the precision and efficacy of these models. Through the data integration layer applied, doctors get a chance to make accurate conclusions, take charge of choices, and, as a result, enhance results for the patients.

Overall, the digital twin architecture includes its physical counterpart, a virtual model, and a data linkage layer, which are put together in such a way as to give digital twins their operating powers and success. A digital twin identifies and symbolically combines real-life, which enables healthcare providers to grasp complex systems, predict outcomes, and real-time optimizations.

Types of Digital Twins

In the healthcare sector, digital twins can be divided into different classes based on their areas of operation and functionality with every class aiming at achieving process optimizations, improving patient outcomes, and increasing efficiency and effectiveness of the operations. These classes are given below.

Patient Digital Twins

Patient digital twins simulate virtual replicas of individual patients which reflect their physical traits, health status, and treatment history in real time. They use data from multiple sources such as EHRs, wearable devices, medical hard copies, genetic or genomic profiles to build personalized models of patients keeping health in mind. Among the features that make up patient digital twins are data about vitals such as blood pressure, medical history, lifestyle factors, and therapy regimens which enable the providers in healthcare to monitor patient health, predict the course of disease, and devise tailored treatment strategies (Hu et al., 2021). A patient digital twin makes this possible by showing the different outcomes of the medications, predicting adverse effects, and prescribing the proper medication dosage that is based on a range of factors like age, gender, genetics, and comorbidities (Erol et al., 2020). Digital twins help healthcare providers take holistic view of patients' health and treatment responses to deliver personalized, precision medicine approaches that help maximize efficacy of therapy and also lower effects of therapy.

Device Digital Twins

The device digital twin makes it possible for the healthcare providers to improve device settings, detect equipment failures, and carry out scheduled device maintenance proactively (Elayan et al., 2021). For instance, device digital twins could track device performance metrics, discover deviations, and alert caretakers of possible problems before they become critical failures such as faulty device operations (Beede et al., 2018). Through the accurate simulation of medical devices in clinical environments, digital twins help avoid patient risks, improve clinical quality standards, and provide healthcare operation efficiencies.

Process Digital Twins

Process digital twins help healthcare organizations collect data, analyse, and improve their internal operations. This computer models use the data obtained from the EHR, administrative systems, operational logs, and workflow diagrams to create complex dynamic models of the healthcare operation processes, covering such areas as patient admissions, laboratory testing, administering medication and discharge planning. Through process simulation, resource utilization, and workflow dynamics, it becomes possible for healthcare organizations to spot delays, inefficiencies, and solutions (Farsi et al., 2020). To illustrate this point, a digital twin technology can play the patient flow simulation in the emergency departments and can identify the flow process problems and then recommend the areas where workflow can be improved to decrease wait times and increase patient throughput (Wang et al., 2021). Through the process of digital twins optimizing healthcare processes, organizations' operations are made more efficient, which contributes to an increase in patients' satisfaction and clinical outcomes.

Facility Digital Twins

At the core of facility digital twin is an exact replica of healthcare facilities where there are designs for the layout, equipment placement, patient flow and environmental conditions to maximize on operation efficiency and patient experience. These digital clones employ data from architectural designs, building systems and sensors, the occupancy and patients' feedback to build virtual environments of healthcare facilities, for instance, hospitals, clinics, and outpatient centres. Healthcare facilities digital twins perform such type of task as simulating both design of the facilities, space utilization, and workflow logistics. This enables the healthcare organizations to optimize the resource allocation, diminish patient wait times as well as enhance clinical productivity (Karakra et al., 2022). As an example, the facility digital twin can be utilized to design different ward layouts, simulate the effect on patient flow and efficiency of staff within that layout among other variables, and recommend the best layout for maximum operational efficiency (Beede et al., 2018). Through facility digital twinning, building design and workflows optimization will be supported by the creation of evidence-based decision-making, cost-effective management, and improved patients' outcomes in healthcare settings.

Digital Twins as a Part of Healthcare Processes

Patient Monitoring and Management

Patient monitoring and management are indispensable parts of contemporary healthcare service. They are not only simple but also essential to ensure patient's needs are met in a timely manner and the patient feel cared for. These days, the implementation of the patient digital twins is one of the key innovations in the area of patient care automation that allows patients to be monitored and managed by healthcare workers more easily. Digital copies of patients (patient digital twins) allow continuous monitoring of vital signs, physiological parameters, and responses to treatment in real time, and, in this way, provide a comprehensive picture of patient health and the possibility to intervene in the machine-human system that can read the necessary signal about health condition.

The patient digital twins' use of sophisticated technology solutions such as wearable devices, sensors, and EHRs is aimed to collect and analyse individual data continuously. Wearable, including smart-watches and fitness trackers, can scan vital parameters like heart rate, blood pressure, and level of activity in real time, thus checking the health conditions of patients (Erol et al., 2020). Health sensors run in tandem with medical devices and at-home systems for monitoring in order to collect additional parameters, like blood glucose level, oxygen saturation, and respiration rate. In so doing, they are making the digital twins of patients even more comprehensive. Integration with the EHR provides medical providers access to historical data, treatment histories, and diagnostic information. Studying past data narrows down the current healthcare situation of a patient to the greater patient's context (Erol et al., 2020).

The advantages which are obtainable through the utilization of patient digital twins in healthcare are numerous. Precise detection of health issues is one the main advantages as digital twins. They can identify minor changes in vital signs and physiological parameters when these changes can be an indication of disease appearance or exacerbation of the existing conditions (Hu et al., 2021). Implementation of patient avatars helps health professionals to notice the issues earlier and hence, the timely intervention prevents complications and improve the patient outcome (Erol et al., 2020). Furthermore, virtual replicas of patients help to design personalized approaches that are customized to the unique features and preferences of individual patients (Hu et al., 2021). Through examination of patient information and effectiveness of medicines, medical personnel can detect what the best treatment strategy is that can make the medicine really effective while it minimizes risks and side effects (Vallée, 2024).

Chronic conditions' remote patient management is another area where patient digital twins are proving highly effective. In this, the technology is being implemented to monitor the health status and treatment adherence of patients having chronic conditions such as diabetes, hypertension, and cardiovascular diseases (Erol et al., 2020). Patient can use wearable devices and home monitoring systems to follow health parameters and medicine adherence while physicians can remotely monitor patient data and intervene whenever necessary in a timely manner (Hu et al., 2021). It is the home-based monitoring system that provides patients with a proactive care plan and prevents multiple visits to the hospital. The patient satisfaction is increased by applying this approach (Erol et al., 2020).

Furthermore, patients' digital twins assist in the continuation of care across different healthcare settings and providers. Through collecting all patient data and treatment histories in a digital format, patient digital twins offer the benefit of facilitating instant messaging between healthcare providers and coordinating their care (Hu et al., 2021). A built-up digital twin will often be dynamic, meaning that it does not stay the same but accompanies patients throughout their healthcare journey, from the primary care visits to the specialist consultations and hospital admissions, ensuring the availability of all the information to the care teams (Erol et al., 2020). The persistent involvement of the patient ensures effective communication, reduces mistakes in medical treatment, and the general standard of the patient care increases.

Medical Device Management

The medical device management is an area that cannot be neglected if healthcare institutions need to achieve the reliability of their services and provide patients with high-quality care. The face of healthcare is now more complex and populated with a large number of medical devices in clinical settings. As a result, physicians and health providers have a lot to do when it comes to monitoring, maintaining, and managing medical devices. In the consequence of the years, using device digital twins has appeared as an effective way to tackle the challenges as it provides real-time insights, predictive analytics and condition monitoring utilities. This allows the management process of medical devices to be more proficient (Tao et al., 2018). Through the utilization of data from sensors, telemetry systems, maintenance records and device specifications, device digital twins will present a combined view of the device condition and status, thus enabling medical care providers to track device performance, determine anomalous conditions, and predict potential problems before they escalate to critical failures (Elayan et al., 2021).

The device digital twins, having the predictive analytics feature as a part of this technology, can allow healthcare providers to foresee equipment breakdowns and perform proactive maintenance in order to minimize breakdowns. The digital twin of these devices employ historical data, a real-time inputs stream, and simulations to predict potential failures and identify root causes of these failures as well as recommend preventive maintenance actions to avoid risks (Beede et al., 2018). For instance, platform digital twins can discover anomalous patterns in the signals produced by the devices, such as those deviating from the baseline parameters or the trends predicting machine malfunctions. After doing so, the twin will notify healthcare providers about the need for corrective actions (Elayan et al., 2021).

By means of regular tracking of the device parameters like temperature, pressure, vibrations and usage patterns, it is possible to perform assessment of device condition and to detect early signs of degradation or malfunction, as well as to generate maintenance alerts as and when required (Karakra et al., 2022). As, for instance, condition monitoring algorithms integrated into device digital twins can read the sensor's data to find out the existing wear and tear in the significant components, predict remaining useful life, and suggest the right maintenance actions so that the device remains in a good performance condition (Elayan et al., 2021). Digital twins also allow for online monitoring of medical tools' performance, which decreases the probability of operational failures, equipment breakdowns, and downtime. All of this prevent disruptions to the clinics' workflow, reduces the risk of adverse events, and enhances the patients' safety (Beede et al., 2018). Similarly, the planned maintenance schedules and proactive interventions through the device digital twin capacity assist in reducing the acquisition cost of devices by extending the devices lifespan, minimize the repair costs, and help in return on investment (Tao et al., 2018).

Drug Discovery and Development

The drug discovery and development remain in the pharmaceutical industry the most laborious and expensive procedure, requiring considerable manual work, trials, and clinical assays to execute successful vaccines. The digital twins' technology has been a remarkable innovation in last couple of years, for the purpose of making the clinical trials and drug development more efficient and quicker. Digital twins conduct virtual screening of drug candidates, pharmacokinetic modelling and simulation of drug interactions which replace the traditional experimental approaches and offer the cheaper and convenient alternatives (Tao et al., 2018).

Digital twins of drug discovery play a major role in virtual screening, where the computer representations are employed to spot drug candidates with the desired pharmacological features. Digital twins in its simulation tools employ molecular modelling techniques like molecular docking, molecular dynamics simulations, and quantitative structure-activity relationship (QSAR) analysis, which can predict binding affinity of drug candidates to target protein and observe their effectiveness (Tao et al., 2018). The digital twins do the job of a shortcut. They make the interaction between the drug molecules and targets' receptors visible, and thus, prioritizing the best candidates for further analysis and validation, and making the drug discovery process faster (Elayan et al., 2021).

Another critical point of drug development where the digital twins are being used as key support is the pharmacokinetic modelling. Digital twins can serve as an ADME (absorption, distribution, metabolism, and excretion) simulations inside the body that can be used to foresee the pharmacokinetic properties of drug molecules and also to optimize dosage regimens (Tao et al., 2018). Digital twins can be individually personalized by integrating patient data collected from the set of demographic information, genetic profiles, and disease characteristics into a physiologically based pharmacokinetic (PBPK) model such that dosing strategies are tailored to the response of the patient's characteristics (Beede et al., 2018). A personalized treatment approach is at the heart of precision medicine as it provides for more effectiveness of the therapy, lesser side effects, and better patient results, eventually leading to better clinical outcomes (Erol et al., 2020).

Treatment Planning

Simulation-based digital twins have completely changed the dynamics of treatment planning in the different specialties such as surgery, radiotherapy, and interventional procedures. These digital replicas of anatomical structures create a realistic environment where healthcare providers can test simulations of patient anatomy and disease progression, along with treatment outcomes in a virtual form. This increases the probability of perfecting treatment options and optimize patient outcomes (Karakra et al., 2022). Digital twins in treatment planning is manifested in various forms such as advanced imaging techniques, for example computed tomography (CT), magnetic resonance imaging (MRI), and 3D reconstruction, which create accurate virtual models of patients' anatomy (Tao et al., 2018). This virtual platform allows surgeons to see complex structures such as the anatomy of an individual, plan surgical approaches, and even identify the structures like nerves and blood vessels that are crucial to the operation (Elayan et al., 2021). Virtual reality simulations can be applied by practicing surgical steps, evaluating possible alternative options in a risk-free environment.

Furthermore, digital twins play an important role in preoperative planning of traditional procedures through simulation, for example in the context of surgery and radiotherapy, as well as interventional procedures, such as cardiac catheterization, endoscopy, minimally invasive surgeries, etc. The digital twin concept allows for reproduction and variation of specific patient anatomy, pathological processes and simulated steps in treatment to allow determination of outcome and best therapeutic option (Tao et al., 2018). Doctors will be able to integrate digital twins into their practice as a tool that allows to consider different treatment options, to review feasibility of interventions, and to prepare a personalized treatment plan to individual patient's needs (Beede et al., 2018). Practicing procedure steps, device simulations, and predicting outcomes of complications help clinicians reduce risks, optimize procedural results, and ensure safety of the patients during interventional procedures (Lukovic et al., 2020).

Healthcare Facility Design

The virtual counterpart of healthcare facilities known as facility digital twin simulates a wide range of features concerning the facility layout, equipment placement, patient flow, and staffing requirements, thus helping healthcare organizations to optimize facility designs as well as workflows for improved patient outcomes and operational efficiency (Karakra et al., 2022).

One of the significant things that facility digital twins are used for is to conduct virtual simulations of a healthcare environment, which is used to assess the effectiveness and safety of layout and design decisions. Using digital twins, relevant CAD 3D models are integrated with GIS data, schedules, and building specifications to create virtual replicas of healthcare facilities (Tao et al., 2018). Through the means of simulating various spacing configurations, furniture arrangements, and spatial relationships, digital twins of health facilities provide a platform allowing healthcare planners and architects to determine the best design options available, identify construction defects, and maximize space utilization for the purpose of achieving a functional and efficient environment (Elayan et al., 2021).

Predictive modelling and scenario analysis outstandingly combined with facility digital twins make it possible for healthcare organizations to look ahead and also to simulate various operational scenarios so that they could optimize resource distributions. The digital twin which relies on historical data, real-time inputs, and predictive algorithms forecasts patient demand, staffing requirements, and equipment utilization under various conditions (Karakra et al., 2022). Role-playing simulations are useful in uncovering operational bottlenecks, testing alternative approaches, and developing and implementing contingency plans which ensure smooth facility performance and rapid response to changing situations (Beede et al., 2018).

The conveniences of the virtual copies of the healthcare facilities in the healthcare facility design and optimization are numerous. Through arranging the layout of the facility and streamlining workflows, medical organizations can improve the quality of patient care and satisfaction by shrinking the waiting time, lessening congestion and redesigning the way-finding (Erol et al., 2020). As an example, facility digital twins can conduct a simulation testing of patients movement through different stages of the facility such as the waiting rooms, examination rooms, and treatment rooms where it can help in identifying the areas of congestion and, thereby, aid in the designing of patient's pathways for improved efficiency.

Other than increased patient outcomes, facility digital twins provide an avenue of using resources properly and hence operational costs are effective in healthcare operations. Through the use of high precision positioning of equipment, efficient workflow, and scheduling of staff, digital twins allow hospitals to optimize resource usage, minimize idle times, and decrease operational costs (Tao et al., 2018). For instance, digital twin can estimate the required staffing levels as per patient demand forecasts, employees' availability, and fitting skills. This can help to provide enough staffing levels to cover patients' needs while cutting labour costs.

Additionally, the healthcare facility digital twins can provide evidence-based decision making and continuous improvement in healthcare facility management. The digital twins help the hospital leaders to monitor essential performance metrics which include operational key performance indicators (KPIs), patient outcomes, and track progress to goals, and the areas where improvement needs to be made which helps in the overall performance of healthcare system (Elayan et al., 2021). Such data-driven way encourages knowledge sharing and innovation, making the culture of inclusive improvements. It helps healthcare organizations to perform better in terms of changing patients' needs, regulations, and external factors.

Conclusion

Digital twins is a revolutionary technology that not only allows for better patient care but also improving organizational efficiency. As such, health-care organizations strive to integrate this technology into their operations to assist in improving patient monitoring, enhancing the well-being of medical devices, treatment planning, developing more efficient designs, it is noted that such endeavours should be coupled with the adoption of lean thinking and other related principles as presented earlier in this chapter. It is only then that the full benefits of digital twins for process improvement can be realized. The long-term impact of this will not only be reduction of overall operational costs but also the improvement of the patient care outcomes and high patient and clinician satisfaction.

References

Beede, E., Baylor, E., Hersch, F., Iurchenko, A., Wilcox, L., Ruamviboonsuk, P., & Phan, T. (2018). A human-centered evaluation of a deep learning system deployed in clinics for the detection of diabetic retinopathy. In Proceedings of the 2018 CHI Conference on Human Factors in Computing Systems (p. 324). ACM.

Dale, B. (1999) TQM: An overview in Dale. Managing quality (3rd Ed). 296 pp. Blackwell, Oxford.

Deming, E. (1986). Out of the crisis. Cambridge University Press, Cambridge.

Elayan, H., Aloqaily, M., & Guizani, M. (2021). Digital twin for intelligent context-aware IoT healthcare systems. IEEE Internet of Things Journal, 8(23), 16749–16757.

Erol, T., Mendi, A. F., & Doğan, D. (2020, October). The digital twin revolution in healthcare. In 2020 4th international symposium on multidisciplinary studies and innovative technologies (ISMSIT) (pp. 1–7). IEEE.

Farsi, M., Daneshkhah, A., Hosseinian-Far, A., & Jahankhani, H. (Eds.). (2020). Digital twin technologies and smart cities (Vol. 1134). Springer, Berlin/Heidelberg, Germany.

Hu, W., Zhang, T., Deng, X., Liu, Z., & Tan, J. (2021). Digital twin: A state-of-the-art review of its enabling technologies, applications and challenges. Journal of Intelligent Manufacturing and Special Equipment, 2(1), 1–34.

Imai, M. (1997). Gemba Kaizen: A common sense, low cost approach to management. McGrawHill, New York.

Inozu, B., Chauncey, D., Kamataris, V., & Mount, C. (2012) Performance improvement for healthcare: Leading change with Lean, Six Sigma, and Constraints Management. Novaces, LLC, Chicago.

Juran, J. (1993). Made in USA: A Renaissance in Quality. Harvard Business Review, July–August, pp. 42–50.

Karakra, A., Fontanili, F., Lamine, E., & Lamothe, J. (2022). A discrete event simulation-based methodology for building a digital twin of patient pathways in the hospital for near real-time monitoring and predictive simulation. Digital Twin, 2, 1.

Lukovic, J., Kim, J. J., Krzyzanowska, M., Chadi, S. A., Taniguchi, C. M., & Hosni, A. (2020). Anal adenocarcinoma: A rare malignancy in need of multidisciplinary management. JCO Oncology Practice, 16(10), 635–640. https://doi.org/10.1200/OP.20.00363

Oakland, J. (2012). Oakland on quality management (3rd ed). Routledge. https://doi.org/10.4324/9780080479781

Saleem, M., Khan, S., Hameed, s, & Abbas, M. (2012) An analysis of relationship between total quality management and Kaizen. Life Science Journal, 9(3), http://www.lifesciencesite.com (accessed August 2012).

Tao, F., Qi, Q., Liu, A., Kusiak, A., & Zhou, L. (2018). Data-driven smart manufacturing. Journal of Manufacturing Systems, 48, 157–169.

Vallée, A. (2024). Envisioning the future of personalized medicine: Role and realities of digital twins. Journal of Medical Internet Research, 26, e50204. https://doi.org/10.2196/50204

Wang, J., Wang, S., Zhang, L., & Zhang, Z. (2021). Digital twin based intelligent risk decision-making system of compressor station equipment. Natural Gas Industry, 41(7), 115–123.

10

The Impact of Blockchain and Digital Twins in the Pharmaceutical Industry

Introduction

Advanced digital and blockchain technologies have highly impacted the pharmaceutical industries. The pharmaceutical industry has undergone an advanced technological revolution to smoothen real-time simulation and analysis inside their operations (Haleem et al., 2022). Advanced digital technology through blockchain has offered significant benefits by decentralizing their system. Digital twins, on the other hand, allow real-time simulation and analysis as physical replica entities. Together, the decentralized, secure, and transparent ledger system assisted by blockchain parallels the integration of digital twins on drug development, manufacturing, personalized medicine, and supply chain management. Therefore, this chapter explores the synergy between digital twins and blockchain technology by examining their critical applications, benefits, challenges, and prospects in pharmaceutical sector.

Introduction to Blockchain Technology

Blockchain technology helps record and manage transactions and data through a distributed ledger system without a central command source. Blockchain technology has spread across various industries beyond Bitcoin through its decentralization nature. Initially, this technology was introduced by an anonymous individual or group called "Satoshi Nakamoto" in 2008 (Dananjaya, 2025). Satoshi Nakamoto's Bitcoin whitepaper explained how blockchain technology would revolutionize the global money system, which does not rely on "central" banks for control (Nakamoto & Bitcoin, 2008). Satoshi did or did not expect his technology to be used across various sectors worldwide. However, what has become hugely transformative is that the technology has gone beyond cryptocurrencies with innovative approaches across different sectors of the world, including the pharmaceutical industry. This is because of its unique features, such as transparency, immutability, and security on systems that require trust and accountability.

DOI: 10.1201/9781003485971-13

Decentralization Aspect

All the mentioned benefits of blockchain technology arise from the aspect of decentralization. The decentralized nature differs from the adopted central nature of operations, where a single entity controls an entire database. Blockchain applies to a different network where peers communicate directly to their peers in a network. The peer-to-peer network allows all participants, called nodes, to have a say on the entire blockchain system (Nakamoto & Bitcoin, 2008). Therefore, the nodes eliminate the need for intermediaries, such as banks, reducing transaction costs and speed. Furthermore, the system's resilience is highly enhanced when services are decentralized since different nodes ensure no single point of failure. If one node goes offline, the blockchain continues through other nodes without disruption.

Transparency

Besides its decentralized advantages, blockchain technology has a transparent way of recording transactions. Through the distributed ledger system, all users in the network can view transactions recorded and verify them to ensure their accuracy (Dananjaya, 2025). In a sector like supply chain management, blockchain technology has been used to enable all participants in the network to view and verify the movement of goods while ensuring transparency and security. These benefits ensure that participants can be accountable and transparent in all their dealings without any party taking advantage of the other. In finance, food safety, and pharmaceutical industries, this level of transparency offered by blockchain is precious.

Immutability

Apart from being decentralized and transparent, Bitcoin's blockchain whitepaper has enabled another essential feature called immutability. Satoshi Nakamoto created a system where nobody can alter or delete a transaction after a transaction is recorded. Immutability allows the creation of cryptographic hash functions, transaction number, date, and amount for each block. Each block has its list of transactions and a cryptographic hash of the previous block (v, 2025). The cryptographic function of each block is an algorithm that cannot be modified since it carries information about the previous block in itself on the chain. If altered, the whole network would collapse. Therefore, the integrity and permanence of the data recorded on the blockchain become reliable and tamper-proof through immutability. In many systems, such as legal practice, medical records, and financial transactions, where data integrity is core, blockchain's immutability benefits have allowed innovative integration.

Security

Another essential aspect of blockchain technology is its security. Using advanced cryptographic functions, Satoshi Nakamoto aimed to create a network where data security is integral. Bitcoin's whitepaper allowed unique digital signatures for every transaction in the blockchain network with public-key cryptography that verifies the transaction's authenticity. The public key ensures that the transaction cannot be altered through a consensus mechanism. Satoshi Nakamoto used Proof of Work (PoW) as the consensus mechanism validating all transactions for Bitcoin. Later, some networks like Ethereum innovatively used different consensus mechanisms such as Proof of Stake (PoS) which required users to stake a portion in the system to be able to validate transitions inside the network before they are added to the blockchain. Major issues affecting the centralized finance system, such as double-spending and fraud (Aquilina et al., 2024), have been fought by mechanisms ensuring that blockchain technology is secure and resistant to such attacks.

Applications across Industries

Many industries have started adopting the network through the features discussed in blockchain technology. What Satoshi Nakamoto created has helped other industries beyond cryptocurrencies to be transparent and traceable. Also, systems adopting blockchain technology have reduced fraud, increasing their authenticity and improving efficiency (Dahal, 2023). For instance, the healthcare industry can ensure patient data is kept securely while seamlessly sharing information among healthcare providers across the system. Additionally, just as in finance, where blockchain facilitates secure and efficient transactions, intermediaries are removed from the systems, increasing data privacy and lowering transaction costs (Aquilina et al., 2024). Creative ways to integrate blockchain have emerged in real estate, focusing on addressing trust, transparency, and security issues. Recently, major economic blocks such as BRICS (Brazil, Russia, India, China, and South Africa) have announced their need to adopt blockchain technology to smoothen transactions between member countries (Zharikov, 2023). Major announcements are expected in Russia in 2024, which chairs BRICS concerning the innovative idea of adopting blockchain technology to fight the centralized finance system controlled by the United States of America.

Future Prospects

Since many industries are on the verge of adopting blockchain, several concerns must first be addressed. One concern about Bitcoin, for instance, was scalability. Blockchain networks use a distributed ledger network that records all the transactions inside. Since the number of transactions keeps increasing, scalable solutions such as sharding and off-chain transactions should be considered for a broader adoption. Another unique challenge may be the interoperability across different networks; since each blockchain network operates in silos, sharing data across different systems may be complex or entirely tricky. Therefore, interoperability standards and protocols must be developed to cater to issues in data exchange. Efforts have been undertaken regarding these two issues. Since blockchain technology has been around for less than 20 years, such a challenge, including regulation, has governments and regulatory bodies trying to find a way of overseeing the network without changing the decentralized nature.

If clear and consistent frameworks for regulation are developed, blockchain technology will transform various industries by transforming traditional processes, enhancing efficiency and fostering trust. In 2024, for instance, the evolving nature of blockchain may introduce ways to address challenges related to regulation (Aquilina et al., 2024) if countries begin adopting cryptocurrencies as a formal way of making payments across governments (Zharikov, 2023).

Overview of the Pharmaceutical Industry

Focusing away from the emerging issues of blockchain technology, the pharmaceutical industry will also be affected by the paradigm shift arising from blockchain technology (Riedel & Velamuri, 2024). Since the discovery, development, manufacturing, and distribution of drugs and medical treatment help the pharmaceutical industry improve health outcomes, innovative ways must be continuously developed. From the complexities across basic research and clinical trials to large-scale production, the quality of life for millions worldwide should be vitally considered.

Discovery and Development

Drug discovery begins with basic research conducted in academic institutions, research hospitals, and pharmaceutical companies. The initial phase, including developing the drugs, explores disease mechanisms and identifies potential therapeutic intervention targets (Chavda et al., 2023). Therefore, researchers can identify new molecular entities and drug candidates through advanced biotechnology, genomics, and bioinformatics to boost drug discovery. After the identification of potential drug candidates, a series of preclinical studies are conducted in vitro (test tubes) and in vivo (animals) to evaluate the safety, efficacy, and pharmacokinetics (Alffenaar et al., 2022) of the components. The series of preclinical studies helps the industry to determine whether a drug candidate has the potential to be effective and safe for human use. If a drug candidate passes the preclinical research, they develop the ability to be effective and safe for human use.

Clinical Trials

If preclinical studies yield promising results, the drug candidate progresses to clinical trials conducted in multiple phases, as explained below.

Phase I

The first phase of clinical trials involves a small group of healthy volunteers or patients and focuses on assessing the drug's safety, tolerability, and pharmacokinetics (Inan et al., 2020). This phase helps determine the safe dosage range and identify potential side effects.

Phase II

These trials involve a larger group of patients and aim to evaluate the drug's efficacy and optimal dosing in the second phase that the drug candidate goes through (Flores et al., 2021). Phase II trials offer preliminary data on the drug's effectiveness to assess its safety on patients.

Phase III

The third phase includes large-scale trials involving hundreds to thousands of patients where trials confirm the drug's efficacy, monitor side effects, and compare it to standard treatments (Khanna et al., 2022). The data from these trials is critical for regulatory approval.

Phase IV

This stage is also known as post-marketing surveillance, where the trials are conducted after the drug has been approved and marketed. As Inan et al. (2020) describe, phase IV trials help gather additional information on the drug's long-term safety and effectiveness, providing necessary data in regard the drug's performance.

Regulatory Approval

The drug development process also involves critical milestones, during which pharmaceutical companies submit a comprehensive dossier with information from preclinical and clinical trials conducted (Alffenaar et al., 2022). The dossier is then presented to regulatory authorities such as the US Food and Drug Administration (FDA) to assess it against required safety standards, efficacy, and drug quality.

Regulatory agencies such as the FDA and European Medicines Agency (EMA) review submissions through an advisory committee and public consultations. The approval process allows thorough inspections of where the drug was manufactured so that all drugs follow Good Manufacturing Practices (GMP) (Aziza, 2021). Therefore, drugs that provide benefit-risk profiles are granted approval to be released into the market.

Manufacturing and Distribution

Next, after regulatory approval, the drug is moved into the manufacturing phase through a collection process where large-scale production of the drug in compliance with GMP standards is conducted. Every batch of the drug is produced during manufacturing and distribution and constantly meets stringent quality criteria. The manufacturing processes after regulatory approval include the formulation of the active pharmaceutical ingredient (API), blending, granulation, tablet pressing/capsule filling, and packaging (Dabrowska & Thaul, 2018). In this step, meticulous control and monitoring to ensure the drug's integrity and effects are maintained.

Finally, the drug goes through its final phase before reaching the client. Distribution involves the logistics of delivering the drug from the manufacturing plants to pharmacies, hospitals, and clinics (Dabrowska & Thaul, 2018). Therefore, an efficient supply chain is needed to manage drug storage and transportation optimally without affecting the quality and effectiveness of the patient.

Challenges in the Pharmaceutical Industry

The pharmaceutical industry faces numerous challenges in developing and delivering new drugs, which are described below.

High Research and Development (R&D) Costs

The pharmaceutical industry's first challenge is developing new drugs, which are expensive and risky. Wouters, McKee, and Luyten estimate that the average cost of bringing a new drug to market exceeds $2.6 billion. This cost includes failed projects and lengthy development timelines (Flyvbjerg et al., 2022). The need for extensive research, complex clinical trials, and stringent regulatory requirements drives high R&D costs.

Stringent Regulatory Requirements

Second, compliance with regulatory standards is essential for ensuring the safety and efficacy of drugs (Aziza, 2021). However, it adds to the complexity and cost of drug development as the standards and requirements vary by region, requiring companies to navigate the global regulatory landscape with more resources and studies.

Emerging Health Threats

Taking many lessons from the recent COVID-19 pandemic, the industry must be agile and responsive to emerging health threats such as the pandemic, antibiotic resistance, and chronic diseases (Goel et al., 2020). Challenges when developing treatments for these evolving threats require rapid innovation, collaboration, and substantial investment by pharmaceutical stakeholders.

Ethical and Social Considerations

Last but not least, pharmaceutical companies face ethical considerations related to drug pricing, access to medications, and the conduct of clinical trials (Petryna, 2005). Balancing profitability with social responsibility is a constant challenge, as companies are expected to consider ensuring that life-saving drugs are accessible to those in need while maintaining financial sustainability.

Importance of Integrating Digital Twins with Blockchain in Pharmaceuticals

Since the pharmaceutical industry experiences significant challenges while ensuring patients have needed drugs and care, digital twins with blockchain technology may hold transformative potential when integrated. The combination innovatively uses real-time, data-driven approaches for an integrity-bound supply chain. Additionally, the cost of the entire process could significantly be reduced, eventually improving patient outcomes (Raj, 2021). Therefore, synergistically, blockchain technology and digital twins may converge to bring a new era of technological advancement and operational excellence in pharmaceuticals.

Enhancing Supply Chain Integrity

Since there is plenty of evidence that the pharmaceutical industry requires an integrity-based supply chain, digital twins could leave a positive influence when integrated. Genuine drugs, safe transport, and optimal storage conditions benefit an excellent patient safety and public health supply chain. Real-time monitoring of products offered by digital twins is needed through every stage in the supply chain (Sahal et al., 2022). Digital twins would solve temperature deviations, delays, or contamination risks through simulation and analysis of the entire drug life cycle.

Additionally, blockchain technology would benefit the system by adding a layer of transparency and security, as discussed previously. Blockchain provides a decentralized, immutable ledger which records every transaction and movement of the drugs while allowing all participants in the supply chain to access the ledger (Sahal et al., 2022). This benefits stakeholders in verifying the authenticity and integrity of the products inside the supply chain. Because those benefits can be accessed at any point, an issue identified is isolated quickly, preventing widespread distribution and ensuring that only safe, authentic products reach patients, especially when a counterfeit drug is detected.

Streamlining Regulatory Compliance

As previously discussed, pharmaceutical companies adhere to strict law requirements through comprehensive documentation to bodies such as the FDA and EMA. Therefore, digital twins and blockchain technology would help streamline this process by ensuring that all data collected during drug development, manufacturing, and distribution is correct, transparent, and accessible to all stakeholders. Additionally, digital twins help with detailed documentation of every step taken when developing a particular drug. The manufacturing process, through digital twins, helps identify and rectify potential compliance issues before escalation. Proactively, this approach enhances compliance by reducing the risk of costly delays or fines (Raj, 2021).

Blockchain technology, therefore, complements what digital twins offer through an immutable record of all compliance-related activities. From laboratory tests to production, every action, including shipping logs, can be recorded on the blockchain to allow regulators to comprehend a verifiable audit trail offered through a simplified review and approval process (Sahal et al., 2022). Moreover, trust between pharmaceutical companies and regulatory bodies will be enhanced in a collaborative effort by all nodes involved inside and outside the regulatory environment.

Advancing Personalized Medicine

Another benefit to be realized is an advanced personalized system of medication. Digital twins boost unique genetic makeup, lifestyle, and medical history with a dynamic, patient-specific model that simulates how different treatments affect an individual. Such models can also be posted by blockchain technology, which helps patients control their data, granting them access where multiple healthcare providers, researchers, and specialists are required. Mechanisms in blockchain technology could also deny the sharing of sensitive genomic data across different research organizations (Raj, 2021). Additionally, a decentralized database of genomic information could boost researchers' efforts to discover new therapies and treatments.

Improving Efficiency and Reducing Costs

For example, in drug development, where digital towns could help simulate the effects of new compounds on virtual models of the biological systems, accelerating the development process could lower the R&D costs during drug manufacturing. Additionally, blockchain technology would enhance efficiency by automating and streamlining various processes. For instance, smart contracts used in blockchain could automate transactions while ensuring execution when only certain conditions are met. Smart contracts would ensure that no intermediaries are involved, hence cutting away administrative overhead, which would otherwise slow the process of transactions (Griggs et al., 2018). Furthermore, a secure and transparent blockchain framework ensures that costly audits and reconciliations are unnecessary.

Enhancing Patient Outcomes

Patient outcomes, the ultimate goal, would also benefit when digital twins are integrated with blockchain technology inside the pharmaceutical industry. The ability to monitor and predict the performance of drugs in real time through digital twins ensures time interventions and adjustments on treatment. Furthermore, personalized medicine, transparency, and traceability provided by digital twins and blockchain ensures patients trust that their medications are genuine and have safely been handled and stored (Raj, 2021). Patients can also receive therapies specifically designed to address their unique health needs.

Addressing Challenges and Barriers to Implementation

This paper has critically evaluated how digital twins and blockchain technology hold significant promise in the pharmaceutical industry. However, challenges in interoperability across different systems and stakeholders from blockchain couples with data-handling problems raised by digital twins arise. The use of innovative technologies also faces regulatory and compliance challenges.

Finally, developing standardized protocols during R&D for data sharing and interoperability is needed when Internet of Things (IoT) devices, cloud computers, and edge devices are made for the pharmaceutical industry. Regulatory and compliance challenges could be addressed if regulatory bodies kept in touch while developing guidelines and standards for use in digital twins (Zoltick & Maisel, 2023) and blockchain. Furthermore, addressing adoption and scalability is essential as it requires collaboration among pharmaceutical companies, technological providers, and other stakeholders. Scalable solutions would be developed and integrated into existing workflows to achieve the full benefits of digital twins and blockchain.

Future Prospects and Innovations

The future expectations of integrating digital twins and blockchain in the pharmaceutical industry are boosted by advancing artificial intelligence (AI) and IoT (Hemdan et al., 2023). Digital twins will drive innovation through such tools for more accurate simulations and predictive analysis where the technologies affect drug development, manufacturing, and personalized medicine. Therefore, more efficient and effective treatments will be developed as digital twins evolve.

Blockchain technology will also evolve, with improvements in scalability, interoperability, and security being explored. Such explorations and innovative ideas will ensure the accessibility and practicality of blockchain in the pharmaceutical industry, enhancing much-required patient data privacy. The industry will benefit from potential innovations in developing decentralized clinical trials with blockchain securely managing the shared data across multiple sites and stakeholders. This approach has positive results on data integrity and transparency for all healthcare stakeholders.

Hopefully, decentralized clinical trials could be supported by blockchain in securely managing and sharing trial data across multiple sites and stakeholders. Beyond improving the efficiency and integrity of clinical trials, decentralized clinical trials would accelerate the development of new treatments (Silva et al., 2024).

Finally, integrating digital twins and blockchain in the pharmaceutical industry could facilitate a more collaborative and transparent data-sharing framework. In such a way, researchers would collaborate quickly and effectively while accelerating the discovery of new medicines and therapies across the entire industry. Continued innovation, evolution, and adoption of digital twins and blockchain will shape the pharmaceutical industry's future in the new era of AI innovation and excellence.

References

Alffenaar, J. W. C., de Steenwinkel, J. E., Diacon, A. H., Simonsson, U. S., Srivastava, S., & Wicha, S. G. (2022). Pharmacokinetics and pharmacodynamics of anti-tuberculosis drugs: An evaluation of in vitro, in vivo methodologies and human studies. *Frontiers in Pharmacology, 13*, 1063453.

Aquilina, M., Frost, J., & Schrimpf, A. (2024). Decentralized finance (DeFi): A functional approach. *Journal of Financial Regulation, 10*(1), 1–27.

Aziza, F. N. Review and comparison of food drug administration (FDA) and medicines and healthcare products regulatory agency (MHRA) on good manufacturing practice (GMP) implementation. *Majalah Farmaseutik, 18*. https://doi.org/10.22146/farmaseutik.v18i2.73520

Chavda, V. P., Anand, K., & Apostolopoulos, V. (Eds.) (2023). *Bioinformatics tools for pharmaceutical drug product development*. John Wiley & Sons.

Dabrowska, A., & Thaul, S. (2018). *How FDA approves drugs and regulates their safety and effectiveness*. Congressional Research Service.

Dahal, S. B. (2023). Enhancing e-commerce security: The effectiveness of blockchain technology in protecting against fraudulent transactions. *International Journal of Information and Cybersecurity*, 7(1), 1–12.

Dananjaya, L. (2025). The digital footprints of Satoshi Nakamoto: A comprehensive analysis of bitcoin forum communications. https://doi.org/10.13140/RG.2.2.36604.65925

Flores, L. E., Frontera, W. R., Andrasik, M. P., Del Rio, C., Mondríguez-González, A., Price, S. A., Krantz, E. M., Pergam, S. A., & Silver, J. K. (2021). Assessment of the inclusion of racial/ethnic minority, female, and older individuals in vaccine clinical trials. *JAMA Network Open*, 4(2), e2037640.

Flyvbjerg, B., Budzier, A., Lee, J. S., Keil, M., Lunn, D., & Bester, D. W. (2022). The empirical reality of IT project cost overruns: Discovering a power-law distribution. *Journal of Management Information Systems*, 39(3), 607–639. https://doi.org/10.1080/07421222.2022.2096544

Goel, S., Hawi, S., Goel, G., Thakur, V. K., Agrawal, A., Hoskins, C., Pearce, O., Hussain, T., Upadhyaya, H. M., Cross, G., & Barber, A. H. (2020). Resilient and agile engineering solutions to address societal challenges such as the coronavirus pandemic. *Materials Today Chemistry*, 17, 100300.

Griggs, K. N., Ossipova, O., Kohlios, C. P., Baccarini, A. N., Howson, E. A., & Hayajneh, T. (2018). Healthcare blockchain system using smart contracts for secure automated remote patient monitoring. *Journal of Medical Systems*, 42, 1–7.

Haleem, A., Javaid, M., Singh, R. P., & Suman, R. (2022). Medical 4.0 technologies for healthcare: Features, capabilities, and applications. *Internet of Things and Cyber-Physical Systems*, 2, 12–30.

Hemdan, E. E. D., El-Shafai, W., & Sayed, A. (2023). Integrating digital twins with IoT-based blockchain: Concept, architecture, challenges, and future scope. *Wireless Personal Communications*, 131(3), 2193–2216.

Inan, O. T., Tenaerts, P., Prindiville, S. A., Reynolds, H. R., Dizon, D. S., Cooper-Arnold, K., Turakhia, M., Pletcher, M. J., Preston, K. L., Krumholz, H. M., Marlin, B. M., Mandl, K. D., Klasnja, P., Spring, B., Iturriaga, E., Campo, R., Desvigne-Nickens, P., Rosenberg, Y., Steinhubl, S. R., & Califf, R. M. (2020). Digitising clinical trials. *NPJ Digital Medicine*, 3(1), 101.

Khanna S, Assi M, Lee C, Yoho D, Louie T, Knapple W, Aguilar H, Garcia-Diaz J, Wang GP, Berry SM, Marion J, Su X, Braun T, Bancke L, Feuerstadt P (2022). Efficacy and safety of RBX2660 in PUNCH CD3, a phase III, randomized, double-blind, placebo-controlled trial with a Bayesian primary analysis for the prevention of recurrent Clostridium difficile infection. *Drugs*, 82(15), 1527–1538.

Nakamoto, S., & Bitcoin, A. (2008). *A peer-to-peer electronic cash system*. bitcoin.org/bitcoin.pdf, 4(2), 15.

Petryna, A. (2005). Ethical variability: Drug development and globalizing clinical trials. *American Ethnologist*, 32(2), 183–197.

Raj, P. (2021). Empowering digital twins with blockchain. In *Advances in computers* (Vol. 121, pp. 267–283). Elsevier.

Riedel, T., & Velamuri, V. K. (2024). Addressing challenges: Adopting blockchain in the pharmaceutical industry for enhanced sustainability. *Sustainability*, 16(8), 3102. https://doi.org/10.3390/su16083102

Sahal, R., Alsamhi, S. H., & Brown, K. N. (2022). Personal digital twin: A close look into the present and a step towards the future of the personalized healthcare industry. *Sensors, 22*(15), 5918.

Sam, S. (2023). Bitcoin in the BRICS: A decade of adoption and economic impact. *Ushus Journal of Business Management, 22*(4), 29–41.

Silva, D. J., Nelson, B. E., & Rodon, J. (2024). Decentralized clinical trials in early drug development—A framework proposal. *Journal of Immunotherapy and Precision Oncology, 7*(3), 190–200. https://doi.org/10.36401/JIPO-23-33

Zharikov, A. (2023). Arbitral award publication by the London Maritime Arbitrators Association: Improving the policy for a greater impact. *Tulane Maritime Law Journal, 47*(2), 245–265.

Zoltick, M. M., & Maisel, J. B. (2023). Societal impacts: Legal, regulatory and ethical considerations for the digital twin. In *The digital twin* (pp. 1167–1200). Springer International Publishing.

Epilogue – Bringing It All Together – DT and Value-Based Care That Is Precise and Personalised

The construct of digital twins is not new. It has been used since the 1960s, firstly by NASA with respect to space initiatives and then later in manufacturing, supply chain management, and the auto industry. More recently, in the last decades, digital twins have revolutionized the German auto manufacturing industry as well as assisted to revive leaner and more effective and efficient manufacturing and supply chain management. To date, the healthcare sector has not ventured into deploying digital twins in healthcare delivery. Only in the last few years have we seen the emergence of the construct in the healthcare literature.

This book sets out to be one of the first to bring the construct of digital twins to healthcare operations and contexts. It did this by specifically focusing on three key parts:

Part I: The Why of Digital Twins/Why Now, where the three chapters:

Chapter 1: Decision-Making in Healthcare and the Rise of Technology and the Impact of the Digital Transformation

Chapter 2: Digital Twins in Other Industries

Chapter 3: The Case for Digital Twins for Healthcare

serve to set the scene and unpack the digital twin construct.

Part II: The What of Digital Twins, which provides the technical backbone of digital twins in the following four chapters:

Chapter 4: From Algorithms to Outcomes: Leveraging Machine Learning Clustering Techniques for Enhanced Clinical Decision Support

Chapter 5: Clinical Decision Support through Federated Learning and Blockchain

Chapter 6: From Algorithms to Outcomes: Leveraging Machine Learning Classification Techniques for Enhanced Clinical Decision Support

Chapter 7: From Perceptron to Liquid Neural Networks: The Evolution of Neural Networks and Their Role in Black Box Modelling for Digital Twins in Healthcare

And finally, Part III: The How of Digital Twins, which describes in three key chapters how digital twins can and should be embraced in various healthcare contexts and operations.

Chapter 8: Digital Twins and Clinical Decision-Making

Chapter 9: Application of Digital Twins in Healthcare Processes

Chapter 10: The Impact of Blockchain and Digital Twins in the Pharmaceutical Industry

It is not possible in one volume to capture the extent and potential of an emerging construct, rather this book serves to fulfill at least two key objectives: (a) to build awareness, and (b) to enable all healthcare stakeholders to gain a deeper understanding and appreciation of how the digital twin construct can assist by leveraging the exponential advances in computing technology to address specific healthcare challenges at a macro-, meso-, and micro-level.

We trust that on the completion of reading this work you, the reader has attained a greater awareness about digital twins for healthcare and simultaneously have gained some appreciation and understanding of how to embrace the construct. Further, we trust that you have more questions now than when you started the book with respect to digital twins, since it is through curiosity and questioning that we can all work to further refine and enhance the role for digital twin to assist in the provision of superior healthcare delivery for everyone, everywhere every time.

The Authors
Professor Nilmini Wickramasinghe
Dr Nalika Ulapane
Dr Amir Andargoli
Melbourne, 1 January 2025

Index